If Heaven Can Wait...

Finding Grace through Alzheimer's

Deedee Sanderson

Published by

GENERAL STORE
GSPH PUBLISHING HOUSE

499 O'Brien Road, Box 415
Renfrew, Ontario, Canada K7V 4A6
Telephone (613) 432-7697 or 1-800-465-6072

ISBN 1-897113-48-X
Printed and bound in Canada

Formatting and printing by Custom Printers of Renfrew Ltd.
Cover art designed and hooked by Lenore Sanderson.

General Store Publishing House
Renfrew, Ontario, Canada

Library and Archives Canada Cataloguing in Publication

Sanderson, Deedee, 1974-
If heaven can wait: finding grace through Alzheimer's / Deedee Sanderson.

ISBN 1-897113-48-X

I. Title.

PS8637.A539I3 2006 C813'.6 C2006-905021-X

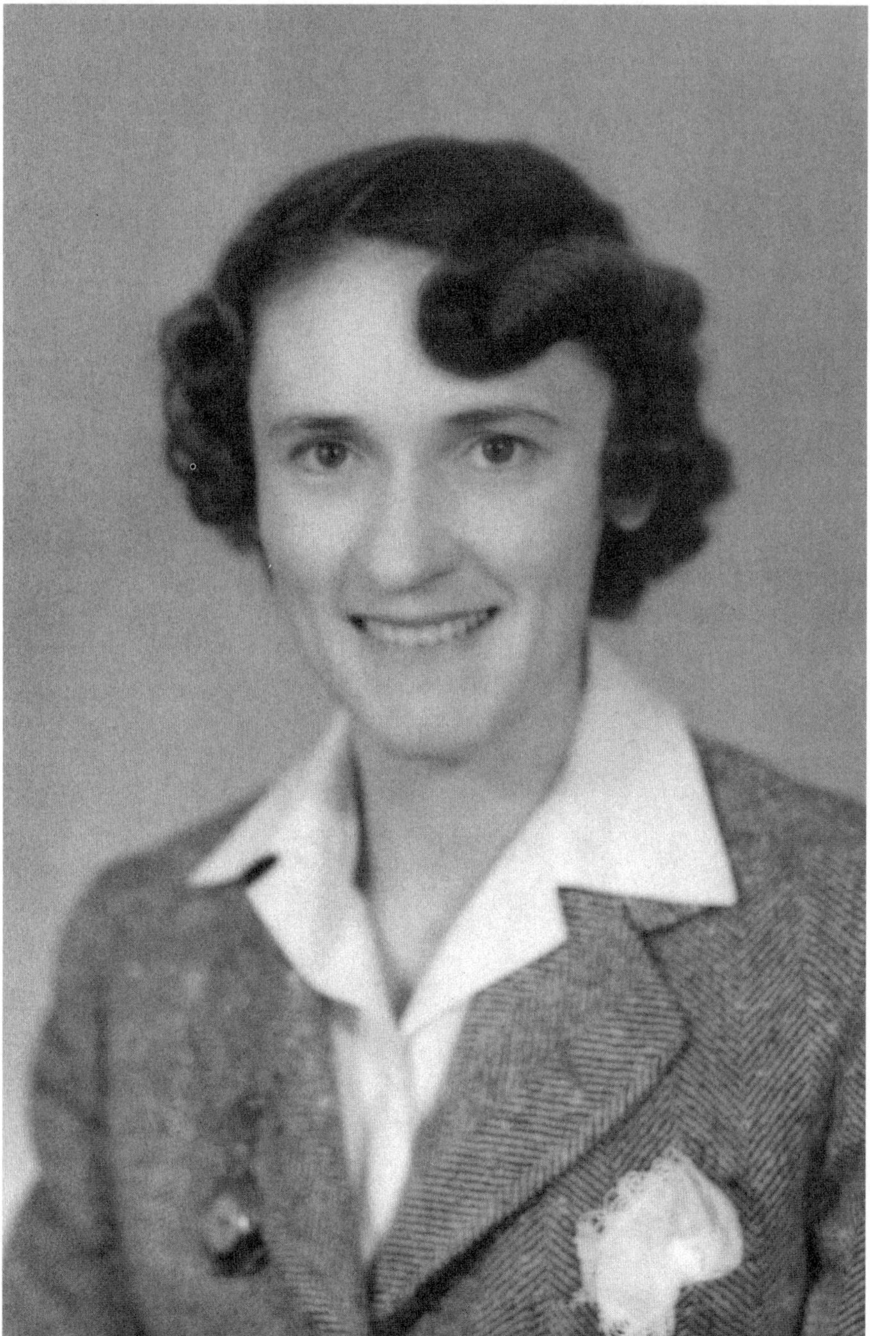

For those who realize that giving themselves to others
is certainly not a sacrifice,
but a gift to grow from.

For those in need who accept help
and allow the circle of life,
this cycle of sharing to occur.

And most of all,
for my granny,
who let her loss of independence be replaced with love and gratitude;
and for all the lessons,
great and small,
we share along the way.

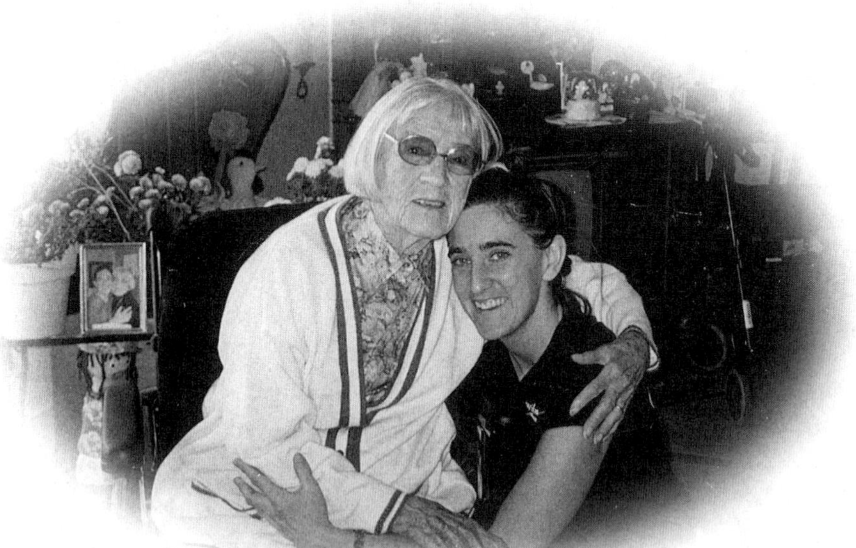

CONTENTS

. . . We Two Shall Wander

It has been brought to my attention that a few details should be clarified before you dive in with us. As this tale goes, it is fitting that hindsight should write the prologue for Granny, who is Lenore, and her granddaughter Heather, who is, at least some of the time, Deedee.

If you were Heather, or Deedee for that matter, you would be kicking yourself for failing to detail Granny's third, "wonderful" bosom buddy. She was Evelyn's sister, Jean, and if you were Heather you would have spent countless hours pouring yourself into the photo album of their Mediterranean cruise, dreaming of a day when you, too, could ride a camel in Morocco and wander the markets in foreign lands—although quite probably wearing far more practical footwear.

If you were Heather, you would have felt admiration for Lenore. This love would have filled you with inspiration and strength. You would not have even realized the impact she had on your life until you had graduated well into adulthood. It is pretty much safe to say that if you were Heather, you would have found yourself in these chapters of your life, perhaps unprepared, but not unwilling, to open your heart in a way you've never felt before.

If you were Lenore, you would give without remembering and take without forgetting. So naturally, if you were Granny, you would thank Heather over and over and over again.

And if you were Heather, you wouldn't mind in the least.

NO SLEEP FOR YOU

"I'm going to die tonight," she said with a smile, a sparkle in her eye. It was a casual statement, not intended to shock or instill pity, but more of a greeting card sentiment . . . "Congratulate me! I'm booking outta here!" No postmarks, no return address. Of course, it's hard to express my own personal sorrow when someone I love is waiting for the gate to open, especially after the long road to get there . . . why? Why has it been locked so long? And who holds the key? What keeps the human soul trapped in an old and tired body? What peace can fill the anguish of a mind tormented with jagged perception and the vanishing ghosts of memories? They haunt the present, these photos of forgotten faces and moments. The glass may be half empty now, but the lips are still wet . . . The memories rise to the surface, but as we reach to touch them they dip under, leaving only the reflection of ninety-two-year-old eyes peering, seeking, and wondering. In the time it takes for them to realize, they vanish, intangible and unattained. Clarity is obscure and variable, entirely undefined.

That day she was as clear as a crystal ball, poignant and poised, articulate and self-assured. "I'm going to die tonight," she calmly reminded me, just in case my memory had failed me. "Let's have a cup of tea; I have a lot to tell you, Heather."

For me, that day had passed like a kidney stone. I think that for Granny it was pretty much an average day, starting with a good scrub from the "bath lady," toast and strawberry jam, half a banana, a can of chocolate Ensure™ over ice, a well-formed BM, and an exquisite ladybug brooch to accent her flowered blouse. She even did the dishes before she reclined onto her perch in her favourite chair to nod off for her morning snooze. With her feet propped atop the footstool she had designed and meticulously hooked, she slowly sank into slumber, as the morning traffic danced through her window.

Myself, I'd settled onto the throne for my own BM (my newly learned acronym), when a scream from the living room sent me hurtling half-dressed (and probably half-relieved) to Granny's side . . .

Fear-filled eyes washed away to extreme joy, sparkling. Giggling, she says, "Hello!"

Okay, let me start that again: giggling, she screams, "HELLO! Did you just arrive from Wilno? Sorry, I was sleeping! LET'S GO FOR LUNCH!"

I wasn't entirely or even slightly sure of what had just happened . . . a bad dream? That seemed, at the moment, the most probable scenario. Her mood was spectacularly gay. Her stamina in high gear, she grabbed her purse, chucked it onto her walker, and headed for the front door.

Now, normally, our excursions begin at the toilet, but not today. We were going out into the April morning with a full bladder and a purse full o' possibilities.

On a good day, she is as tipsy as a roly-poly clown pin, the kind that pops back up when you tip it over. It was a challenge to convince and assist her to put on a coat before gallivanting into the early spring air. Her always dignified self took the time to tuck the hip pouch that housed an antibiotic pump under her pants. The drugs were treating the osteomyelitis, a bone infection that had set into her fractured elbow, yet another drama that began in high-heeled shoes and led to the acute-care floor of a seniors' residence. A story I will tell you later . . . timelines are hazy here . . . I will try and keep on track for all our sakes, but bear with me if I take us down too many roads at once.

Her sense of humour sparkled as she winked and said, "I'M PREGNANT," gesturing to the awkward pouch that pumped massive doses of meds three times daily into her frail body. That damn thing certainly made life interesting for the five-week run, a medical necessity that saved her life, or at least her right arm, and created practical mayhem for both of us.

Back to the story . . . our lunch was light and cheery. We discussed feelings and the newly arrived birds, explaining to the waitress that Granny was turning ninety-three next week and that she was indeed pregnant, an acceptable excuse for the bulge under her pants. In Granny's eyes it is far more respectable to be expecting a child than be construed as fat or on medication. A small white lie kept Granny from being self-conscious and kept the waitress guessing and grinning. We tend to do that to waitresses—keep them grinning, that is.

We returned home with the lucky day attitude, as "WE HAVE NO DISHES!" is a fine excuse for dining out—which she'd do every day, every meal, if she could. She likes to feed people—likes to provide the food. And she likes to go out. Three birds with one stone made Granny satisfied to go back to the house. Tuckered out, both of us, I convinced her to have a snooze on the couch, a momentous achievement on my part; in five months she'd always refused to lie down in the daytime to rest, preferring catnaps in her throne overlooking the street.

I took the opportunity to pay a few bills and delve into my income taxes. I have to admit that I was getting pretty damn tired. My role as primary caregiver was at times gruelling, full of emotion and lack of sleep, but evenly keeled with the beauty of sharing this time with such a vibrant and wonderful woman, a woman who I can honestly say changed my life every time I saw her in the past thirty years.

To make my whole situation here even more interesting and undoubtedly stressful, I'd applied for more care hours from our community care provider. I was struggling to complete all the errands in the fifteen hours per week allotted for personal-care time my granny had, let alone get out for a walk or a rushed coffee with a friend.

I was in between sink or swim—I think it's called treading. Treading . . . going nowhere but still breathing . . . not bad, all things considered. To make a long story short, I had finally found a lawyer to help me through the red tape of the appeal process. He was and is a sympathetic gentleman who had a background in matters of dealing with the Ministry of Health and Long-Term Care, the folks who pull the strings in matters such as ours.

Back to our story, I was conversing on the telephone with Ernie when her own scream woke Granny from slumber. I watched in horror as her legs lifted from the couch, arms locked in front like a zombie, eyes rolling and teeth clacking. I hung up on the councillor and held Granny as the shaking passed through her like an earthquake.

"I'M NOT GOING TO THE HOSPITAL!" She is always very direct. "DON'T TELL GEORGE!" George is her son, my father, and she never wants to worry him.

"I'm going to die tonight." And the laughter—she laughed like there was no tomorrow, and why not? There might not be a tomorrow, so we laughed together, hard and from the heart.

After a few moments, she had no recollection of the incident and was good to go. Better than good—she was stoked. I was her shadow as she zipped around the house in a flood of acute memory. "I made that . . . I did that . . . I paid twenty dollars for that . . . and oh boy, we'd better organize this drawer and tidy that closet!" And "Listen, Heather, my Will is complete. My son will inherit everything . . . but when he has the auction . . . you should bid on the china. It is lovely china, and you'll probably get a good deal on it." Wink. Wink. Nudge. Nudge.

That brings us to our evening tea, and the recollection of the three fur coats in her closet, which incidentally were no longer there. Two of the coats had somehow disappeared at some point in 2004 and the third I had given to her best friend, who would still be able to walk under the weight of the multitude of mink. There was no time to explain this situation to her before she was off again, to show off her furs to me.

I haven't yet mentioned that Granny is profoundly deaf and has unfortunately lost her ability to lip read. We communicate through writing. I write, she speaks, a laborious means of interacting, especially when someone's on a dementia high and basically running with his or her walker. "I'm going to die at home," she states. She is always direct.

With that, we're off to take inventory of her furs. She gets stuck at a closed door, me behind, Granny, and then the walker . . . a traffic jam of sorts in the Iris Street hall. I slink around to reach the knob, pondering the reaction she would have when she sees that all her furniture is gone . . . replaced with my stuff . . . after all, I had just arrived this morning for a visit.

That is when the third seizure hit. I was trapped from Granny by the walker. However seizures seize, she fell over backwards, like a plank in the wind. Her head was first to klonk on the metal of the cold air exchange grate. The blood began to pool into the room. I was torn between being at her side and finding the phone. If she was about to die, I wanted to be by her side.

Being alone in these situations is pretty freaking INTENSE.

The 911 response was fast. She was lucid after a time of screaming and moaning. Sideways notes: *Where does it hurt? I love you.* She continually reminded the paramedics that her son was to inherit everything and that she'd upholstered all the cushions in the living room and paid twenty dollars for the wood frames. Yes, she'd made the pillows, too.

It was 8:30 or 9:00 and I was totally exhausted. The prior night was pretty much sleepless for me due to the constant need to urinate—her, not me—and the constant raging ringing in her ears, both side effects of the liquid antibiotics; not to mention the occlusions in the line of the machine. The high-pitched squeal of a transport truck reversing alarmed me that the line was pinched closed somewhere between the pump and Granny. Needless to say, I was up more times than I could count; no need to even try counting, really.

How, I ask, do you keep a sleeping Alzheimer's patient from re-bending her arm? I "MacGyverred" a contraption with a tensor bandage and ruler; it worked for about half an hour until Granny removed the ruler . . . "Why would I have a ruler stuck to my arm? How odd."

Anyway, that was the night before, and the night before that, and the one before that. Hell, it was like that for most nights in the later part of the antibiotic period. The night I'm talking about now was the night we ended up at the Queensway Carleton Hospital. I'm running on adrenalin, and she's under observation.

Our notes would have looked something like this: "*They are going to glue your head up. Try and keep your arm straight. I love you. No, no. I want to stay. I will stay and help you. Please let me stay to help you. Try and keep your arm straight. Yes, you paid your taxes.*"

She's "under observation," yet nobody sees the several seizures that she endures while awaiting the crazy-glue surgery. Diagnosis: I must be overreacting as a concerned granddaughter, so with a couple of potassium capsules in her belly, they transport her home around one a.m. I was to wake her every hour (lovely) in case of concussion. I race ahead to clean up the blood and hopefully have a few minutes to put my feet up before I have to change her from her bloody pajamas and try to get her settled into bed . . . I even set the alarm for one hour. One hour? A little voice in my head whispered, "No sleep for you."

Ahhhh . . . I will always remember what my pillow felt like for the time I had, horizontal, my bed a sanctuary, my head reeling but slowing down. Granny was fervently talking in her sleep . . . I was up and down to check . . . before the alarm even went off . . . is she calling to me? What is she saying? Is she in pain?

I must have nodded off because her shriek for help ripped me out of somewhere. Another seizure had gripped her and flung her from bed. She was half on the floor, twitching, her right shoulder jammed between the mattress and the bed rail. Vomit on the pillow and the floor. Lovely! She was screaming in pain and yammering nonsense. After several failed attempts, I finally got her freed of the bed rail and lying flat on her back, in a pool of puke. Once again, lovely. Lovely.

She obviously wanted off the floor. She is not only direct but also very determined. To no avail, of course; she was stuck on the floor.

We wait for the paramedics there, together on the floor, about ten feet from where we lay a couple of hours before. Her strength is gone and my nerves are shot. "Don't tell George," she reminds me. Zippity-doo! We're off to the hospital for the second time in our long day.

No sleep for you, my little voice confirmed. *No sleep for you.*

"SOMEBODY'S STOLEN MY CHEQUEBOOK!"

Prior to the time that I moved to Ottawa to care full time for Granny, I would go once a week to help her out. I would visit for the night and go for groceries, run errands, make appointments, go to appointments made, take her out on the town, and assist in housekeeping duties. I was aware of her memory loss and medical conditions and was concerned with her living alone; however, the reality of the situation was: Granny was deemed competent to make and carry through with any decisions regarding her life. She wanted to stay at home and was legally allowed. Shine on!

The only person, I think, to change this status would be her doctor, who told me flatly, "If you put her in a home, she will die of depression."

As the Power of Attorney for her personal care, I was getting a lot of calls from hospitals announcing newly broken bones from weeding dandelions and moving television sets. Really. Stubborn and determined and well-dressed. Independent and not aware of her own limits.

The independence part really made it hard to help her. I had to do it without her knowing. So, we'd go for groceries, and I'd choose all her favourite foods. When the time came for me to return home for work, she would attempt to send me off with everything we'd purchased, saying, "I'll just take the bus and pick up groceries tomorrow." She was, in her eyes, fully capable of taking the city bus, with a broken wrist and a cane, to pick up a week's worth of groceries, in stylish red heels to match her summer coat.

You can ascertain, things were slipping. The bank ladies were always so relieved to see that I came to the bank with Granny. It turns out that she would come often to withdraw money alone, just tempting the waiting mugger who overhears the sweet old lady, her pearls sparkling as she steps up to the wicket and screams, "I WANT A THOUSAND DOLLARS!"

"**A THOUSAND DOLLARS**!" she'd confirm, a little louder, just in case the teller was hard of hearing.

I'm sure they watched in horror as she'd bid them good day, yell, "I'M LOADED!" and proceed to recount her cash as she waits for the bus to return home or go to Sears.

Granny was never a big spender—on herself, that is. For friends and family, money was never an object, but a means to please and show her love. Even now, in the throes of Alzheimer's, her purse is a talisman. It can buy things, pay for things; it holds Kleenex, a photo of George, and about five pounds of stuff. It is too heavy for her to easily manoeuvre with, throwing her off-kilter as it sways with her gait. Waking in the hospital from comas or semi-comatose conditions, her first thoughts and words have been: "I want to go home," and "Where's my purse?"

At one point she was suffering from edema, a symptom of congestive heart failure, and the infected ulcers were bursting on her legs; she didn't have the energy to transit to the mall. As a shopaholic, she went a little crazy and purchased a large monetary sum of jewellery from a door-to-door saleswoman, which to me is taking advantage of an old lady, but I guess we all get our just deserts.

This peddler must have gotten the shock of her life when Granny realized that "someone has stolen my cheques!" and was forging her name. The bank was quick to react—they weren't going to have anyone taking advantage of this sweet old lady. We charged the woman with fraud. It was all a bit of a comical oops! when we later realized the misunderstanding: Granny had signed the cheques with her *left* hand, due to the broken wrist. High drama with a hint of karma; perhaps this seller will think twice before selling old ladies necklaces without receipts—or even *with* receipts, for that matter. It was our eye-opener; well, mine and the bank's, but not Granny's. She never admitted to ever writing the cheques; blind pride is what that's called, and if that keeps her happy, then that is what she can believe. A little grace goes along way when you're ninety-two.

UNDER OBSERVATION

Once again, we were under observation, and no one saw anything. I think that that is an oxymoron and should be lyrics in a song.

I waited by her side and called out to the nurses when the seizures hit . . . always too late they would arrive, only witnessing the laughing spells. Hallucinations started—Granny, not me. Finally a close-by doctor saw a seizure and stated, "She's having seizures" in a matter-of-fact tone, as though he were the first to realize this. Tests. Drugs. A blur, a blur.

Indeed, at this point I was wise enough to reach out to our angel in disguise, a wonderful woman named Cheryl who worked for a senior care companion agency. This was my only oasis over the long winter as an alternative care provider—my only key to freedom from the house, apart from Betty, whom I will tell you about later.

Emotionally and physically drained, it was a relief to have Cheryl arrive to hold a frightened and distressed Granny's hand, and a tired and frazzled Granddaughter's hand, too. (Cheryl has gotten to know Granny quite well since her first evening with Granny, New Years' Eve 2005—my first night off, first *hours* off, since Granny had returned home.) Her tears flowed freely with mine, and I felt like my soul sister had arrived at the hospital. Strangely enough, I had had a powerful dream back in January about Cheryl and myself, a vague dream of two women crying; our tears of release, joy, and sorrow blended as we melted together with emotions into one bright light. I'm sure on some level Cheryl knows how important her connection is to Granny and me, but not the actual height of gratitude I feel inside myself. I am amazed at how a total stranger can have become such an important crutch and a dear friend.

With Cheryl comforting a screaming and hallucinating Granny, I got a little downtime and collapsed onto the lawn to cry my eyes out. It was almost lunchtime the next day from the first seizure. I had been awake for over thirty hours in crisis mode. Cheryl stayed with us as the seizures got stronger and more regular. We held her down as the anti-seizure medication burned into her veins. Lots of insects were crawling on the ceiling and curtains. We tried to keep her eyes closed so she could relax in entomology central. They administered Dilaudid, a morphine derivative to alleviate the pain of the other medicine. At that time, test results confirmed that no stroke had occurred; the seizures were due to scarring on her brain. That is due to the Alzheimer's disease—the brain gets damaged and repairs itself with scars; scars that short-circuit thoughts and electricity.

The rest of the day is extremely foggy for me . . . I may have followed the hospital bed to her room . . . I may have even eaten dinner . . . I did eventually get some sleep, chased home by the nursing staff to sleep beside the phone and wake up to Tim Horton's coffee at the Queensway Carleton Hospital, my new home away from home.

OUT ON THE TOWN

We're out on the town . . . Granny wants to go for coffee . . . she always wants to go for coffee, and quite honestly I'd rather go for coffee than go for dinner. Going for dinner is a challenge at best for a moderate eater. I'm guessing it's due to the provider nature of my granny that purchasing and watching the consumption of food creates a great euphoric high in her. She says always with wide arms, "ORDER SOMETHING BIG!" and is profoundly and personally offended if the pile of food is smaller than your head. It is equally disheartening for her to see uneaten food left on your plate when you can't possibly eat another bite. She, on the other hand, will eat only two bites and proclaim, "I'M TOO EXCITED TO EAT!" and gets the rest "PACKED UP FOR LUNCH TOMORROW," yet another science experiment for her fridge to grow. Then we ask for a souvenir; if they have nothing to sell, the waitress finds something to give her to remember that particular outing. We usually put masking tape on the bottom with the date and she makes me sign it, like I made this object appear into her life. It is as if without the date and name the object were nothing but a question to nag her mind.

Which is sort of like the Polaroid photos we take. They, too, must be immediately labelled, even before they develop. Granny has two Polaroid cameras. I found them in the closet where the furs once hung, with about ninety-six sweaters from Sears. On a brainwave to solve the "WHO'S COMING OVER?" stress, I got film for the old camera and we take pictures of nearly every visitor—always a thrill for Granny—a touch of magic in our world.

They say a picture's worth a thousand words and I'd say they're worth a lot more than that. If you have Alzheimer's, you would never get to the thousandth word and remember the 400th, but a picture—ahhh . . . yes, those friendly faces, a "*This* person is coming over" instead of a "WHO?"

Anyway, we're out on the town, out for coffee at the Second Cup. I've decided to introduce Granny to *haute* culture, well at least urban culture and not Tim Horton's. We've sort of even dressed up; this is pre-walker times, so Granny still has control of her footwear (stylish low patent-leather heels). Her twenty-year-old photo-grey glasses are darkened from the sun. She looks rather hip—red's her favourite colour and she wears it well. She always tells me that red is my colour, too, perhaps because she likes it so much.

We order lattes—"HOW SWISH!" she'd have said, with all the fancy sprinkles. She had a muffin and I had date square . . . any excuse to feed.

Here's the scene: me and Granny in the café, full of, I daresay, serious professionals, apart from a table of giggling girls drinking strong coffee and phoning boys on their cells. We're busy writing and reading and talking and listening—probably curious behaviour for the outsider looking in. They can clearly hear Granny's shrill and excited exclamations but cannot perceive the other side of the conversation. Her glass-shattering squeal breaks the din of chatter. It may have even stopped the music, blowing the speakers with its decibels. She leans into me, to whisper behind her well-defined fingers. Due to the horror of her discovery she doesn't whisper but screams full force into my ear, "THIS MUFFIN'S MOULDY!"

It was a moment that stopped the clocks like a movie put on pause. No one moved or spoke. Muffin eaters everywhere stopped chewing and considered spitting and rinsing. Of course, the manager heard her proclamation and rushed to replace the muffin with a mould-free one, not that she had an appetite at that point. "I'M TOO EXCITED TO EAT!"

Still on her wits' edge, she leaned over to whisper, but once again screamed into my other ear, "NO WONDER THEY CALL THIS THE SECOND CUP!"

We certainly didn't take that muffin to go.

And we also never went back.

"THINGS ARE MAKING SENSE NOW"

Things ARE *making sense now.*
Sometimes thoughts just poof!
Sometimes, just nothing can make sense.
But I know I am upset about something.
I can't remember what it is!
It's upsetting!
It's upsetting to me not to remember.
Now I'm upset because I can't remember.
Why am I upset?
I just can't put my finger on it!
And it's driving me crazy!
I KNOW *that I'm upset about something.*
Oh wow! WOW!
Look at those lovely flowers!
I love flowers!
They smell so wonderful!
I love flowers, especially roses.
Who, me?
No, I'm not upset about anything.
I love flowers.
Flowers are wonderful!

WAITING FOR PEACE

Eating has been a major issue for us. It's just sort of mellowed out since the late-June stroke or whatever happened in medical terms. Whatever it was, it caused a lot of diarrhea and a semi-comatose condition, for a spell. "This could be it," Dr. C warns . . . and rightfully so . . . I've learned by now that any moment could be it, especially if you're ninety-three. But for someone with as much gusto and determination as my granny, I can imagine she would never die if she were sick. She'd get better first and then die. Really, I'm sure the only way she would actually let go would be if she were totally in peace, never giving up in a fight.

I saw this first-hand at the Queensway Carleton Hospital during the seizure stay; it was a really beautiful moment that will be with me until my memory fails me, perhaps even longer.

Once admitted to her private room on I think it was the fourth floor, she was either asleep or in another world and time zone. I'm pretty sure it was a drug-induced stupor . . . an open-window brain with a time-warp button. Sometimes she was present and lucid, but her words were all wacky. She thought I was crazy for not understanding. Sometimes, though, she'd hear herself and laugh at the words. Hear herself? Hmmm . . .

Anyway, we are here in room 406, where scarring due to Alzheimer's caused misfires in her brain, where later tests showed a stroke did occur in her right frontal lobe. Her kidneys were failing. To be perfectly frank, she hadn't had a shit in five days. She'd quit drinking and would pull restlessly at the IV and oxygen tubes. The unprocessed liquids due to kidney failure were filling her up like the Michelin Man. Her lungs were gurgling, each breath taking great effort. She coughed and coughed under the water of herself, an agonizing sound to bear for hours a day, let alone endure as the breather of the harrowed breaths.

I put in sixteen-hour days, until my sister would arrive. I wanted to be with Granny as much as possible—she was confused and scared. Anna was coming daily after work, partly to keep me sane, I think, but mostly to see her neighbourhood granny. We pushed the nurse button often and waited and waited . . . they were busy . . . We waited sometimes twenty minutes, an agonized and impatient time. We would laugh nervously and I'd even admit that I might have let the laughter get a little out of control at times. I was pretty much tired of crying. We must have sounded like two freakin' lunatics, but I'm sure it helped; the laughter, that is. Granny wouldn't have wanted us crying, that's for certain. It would have pissed her off to have anyone feel sorry for her, even in this near-death state.

I was alone with her a lot. I had to remind the staff to roll her over—I couldn't do it alone but was quickly learning the tricks of the trade. She had a bedsore on her tailbone, her skin breaking down from the pressure of her unmoving body.

She wakes up and is right there for the first time in a long while. She looks straight into my eyes. "Heather, I'm scared."

"*EVERYTHING IS FINE*" I write big, in Sharpee™ marker. Her reading is slow. She rereads it several times, eyes clicking over the letters. She nods.

"Is everything looked after?" peering eyes.

"EVERYTHING IS LOOKED AFTER," I confirm and nod.

"Heather, there are lights everywhere."

"*IT'S OK. GO TO THE LIGHTS. IT'S PEACEFUL THERE.*"

"Okay, Heather." She closes her eyes and an angelic aura spreads across her face. Eyes open, "Can I go to the lights?" I smile and nod. Another few moments of peace pass and she says, "Everything is looked after . . . I can go to the lights."

She actually smiled then, and pulled me down to get a kiss. We look at each other for a long while. She nods again, and closes her eyes in peace.

Then, a coughing spell zaps her into pain and reality and instead of passing over she's caught in the violence of drowning in her own body.

I can only hope that her peace will, at some point, be long enough to let go. That is my hope and my prayer, for Granny to have a little peace, a long enough moment to escape the pain and suffering she is enduring.

With wet eyes and nose running, I push the nurse button and wait.

That's what we do at the hospital—wait.

We wait for meds, doctors, nurses, care relief, and perhaps the Grim Reaper, although we'll soon see that he is waiting, too—this is not Granny's time to be taken from the earth. The angels are watching over her patiently. They are the only ones not waiting for anything. They are simply there, watching over us with warmth and assurance.

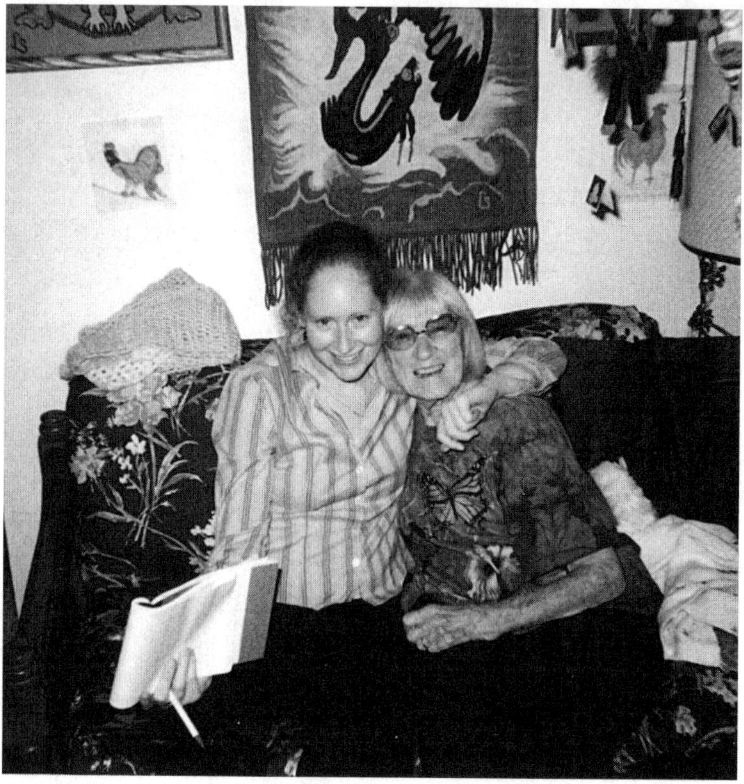

Anna and Lenore

STICK IN TILL YOU STICK OUT!

So it wasn't the April stroke that changed the food habit, it was the June one, if that's what happened in June; your guess is as good as mine, or even her doctor's, for that matter. If in these times in question, I actually took the time to journal Granny's behaviours, reactions, and side effects, then I guess I would have time. Indeed, another brilliant puzzle thought for a song: "If I had time, I would have time." Reality, however, sets in and I can only reflect on changes in hindsight; retrospective analysis.

Prior to late June, Granny would only eat when you ate and what you ate, literally bite for bite. She'd say, "DO YOU WANT A COOKIE?" meaning: "I want a cookie . . . have a cookie and I'll have a cookie." So many unwanted cookies I have consumed or carefully hidden up sleeves or in couch cushions . . .

I'm not sure what strokes do in the brain; well, physically I understand the ramifications but psychologically I am slowly learning. The June Thing, which is not a proper title but it will help keep all these different situations defined, must have short-circuited this *I eat bite for bite* syndrome, and now Granny will eat pretty much whatever you put in front her, even if it's not ice cream.

That's not to say she doesn't get pleasure from watching others eat anymore, but now she doesn't force you to eat everything she eats. This is a relief for me, to say the least, and one behaviour I certainly don't miss.

Granny's grandmother used to say, "Stick in till you stick out!"—an expression that Granny still used frequently, even daily, until this June. An expression that enforced the rule of the roost: eat until you're sick. And enjoy it. Every bite. Have another cookie!

I'm certain that living through the Depression invigorates one's need to feed and provide. If it will pleasure a little old lady to watch me consume a cookie, I'll mow down on a cookie, or at least pretend to—and pretend to enjoy it: "Delicious! Thank you for the cookie!"

"My pleasure, Heather, my pleasure!" Her pleasure, really. Her pleasure is mine.

Stick in till you stick out!

Evelyn

I can only imagine the social bug that infected my Granny throughout her lifetime. Company was always welcome, encouraged, and expected. Her homemade cookies always ready, finely displayed on her beautiful china, the dishes I am to bid on at the auction. Her teapot rarely cooled down between guests, she always pre-heated it with scalding water to ensure only the best Tetley was served. "Strong enough to stand your spoon up in it!" she'd brag. "It's a fine brew! Have another cup!"

She had so many acquaintances and some dear, dear, friends—most of whom are pushing up daisies now and might only be a flash of recollection for her . . . remembrance sparked by a photo, an object, or a hallucination. She had three "best friends" that stand out for me from the throngs of people who faithfully visited, wrote, and gifted her with chocolates for Christmases and birthdays. She never forgot them, until recently when the Christmas cards would arrive, and she would stare puzzled at them and say, "Who's that?" Sometimes it would upset her but I think that all in all she is still flattered to receive countless cards over the Christmas season.

Evelyn was a woman I would have wished to meet—do wish I'd met—but feel I know through stories told by my father and Granny. I'm sure she is still watching over Lenore and is an invisible cloak of strength and comfort.

In our lifetimes we are blessed when someone steps up to bat for us. Evelyn was a rock in the many shaky times my granny endured. Evelyn endured, is enduring, and will always be endured in the heart of Lenore. I think that she carried Lenore through the roughest waters of her life . . .

A thing that is little spoken of, and probably never accepted by my granny, was the horrible reality of fearing for her life as her husband, that man she loved with every ounce of her being, even now in the present day, beat her with open hands and fists. And if living through it once, twice, however many times weren't enough, she got to relive the betrayal half a century in the future.

It's funny how time can criss-cross into the now, the past more real than the present moment. I was a fly on the wall that winter night when her dreams—nightmares, more correctly—manifested into reality.

"YOU'RE GOING TO KILL ME!" She trembled as she yelled. I sat straight up in bed. *What*?

"YOU'RE GOING TO KILL ME ONE OF THESE TIMES!" I slunk to her bedroom door. She was half sitting, eyes wide and staring, hands up, on guard, blocking the strikes that assaulted her space. "NO! NO! NO!" she screamed. "GET OUT! YOU'RE GOING TO KILL ME!"

I was dumbfounded, to put it mildly. She was neither awake nor asleep. She was looking, but her eyes were dancing with a different light, a light from somewhere else, more directly from another time. All I could do was watch the scene . . . how does one take part in a hallucination? For certain, I didn't want to upset her any more than she already was, as she fought for her life.

"THAT'S IT! IF YOU WON'T LEAVE THEN I'LL SLEEP ON THE COUCH!" she stormed. With that, she threw her blankets onto the walker. With pillows teetering atop the pile she screamed, "I CAN'T TAKE THIS ANYMORE!" and pushed past an invisible husband, elbowing her way by to get to the sanctity of the sofa. I realized that I must intrude on this reality, mostly because she'd never make it to the couch with the precarious load of linen, wool, and quilt.

She sees me at the door, I am there to her. Whew! I am there but I'm not me, I'm Evelyn and I'm a welcome sight to Granny, to Lenore, to a poor woman who's frightened and weary. I am glad to be Evelyn in that moment and probably, in any moment in my granny's eyes for that matter. It gives me great honour to be you, Evelyn. I held Granny for a long time. When our tears subsided and she could see again to read, I assure her,

"He's gone.
He won't be coming back.
He can't hurt you anymore."

Eventually I get her settled into her safe little bed. "He can't hurt me anymore? . . . He can't hurt me anymore," she mumbles as she starts to doze off. Of course there was a final, gracious "Thank you" that escaped her lips; "Thank you, Evelyn, thank you."

Thank-yous come in threes from Granny, and from me, too. I thank Evelyn in her place in Heaven—Evelyn who lived down the street from my granny and spent most of her spare time with Lenore and George. It was Evelyn who presumably took all the photos of this mother and son; and Evelyn who knit all George's knickers, socks and sweaters. And quite devastatingly, it was Evelyn who was struck dead at the end of Lenore's laneway by a passing car. I don't know what season it was, what year it was, or even the time of day. I don't know if Evelyn was coming or going. It is not a moment I ever want to recall in my granny. It is a moment that could easily break the heart and will of any best friend or young man who had spent years with such a wonderful woman.

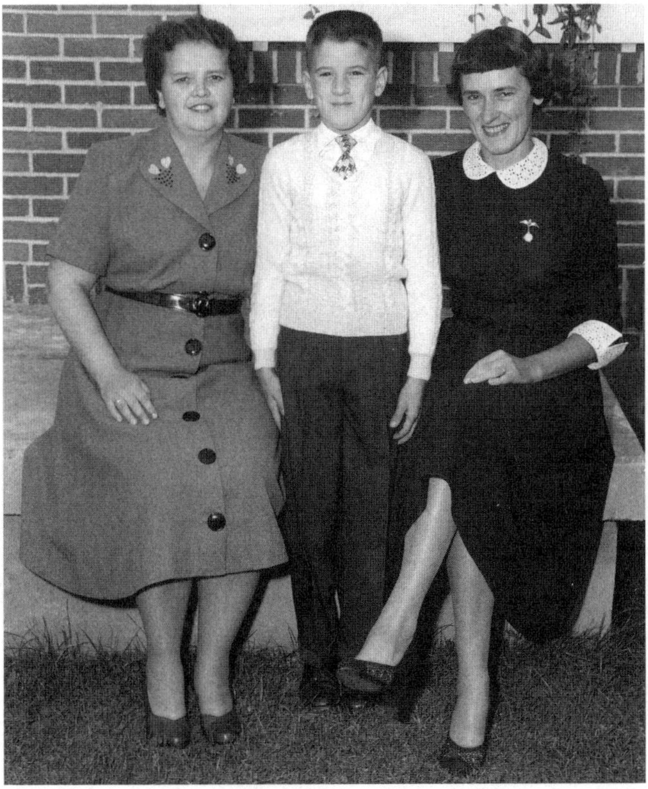

Evelyn, George, and Lenore

Granny really never spoke of it, merely matter-of-fact statements like, "Evelyn was killed at the end of my laneway." Period. I assume that it's a deep wound that someday may surface and even subside; perhaps she will let go of its pain before she is carried to the grave. In my heart of hearts—in my soul, I suppose—Evelyn is and will be waiting for her dear Lenore on the Other Side, arms open and smiling with a pair of size seven hand-knit socks and oven-hot apple pie.

THE WATERFALL

My granny has told me a lot of stories, many of them twice. If she told them to me twice, she's told me them several times into infinity. As her memory fails, the stories get fewer and fewer but her favourites are repeated . . . I'll watch with laughing eyes—oh yes, this story again, still anticipating the climax, like rereading a good book.

Take for instance her story of the California mountain. Once again, a "fashion-plate" Lenore is "dressed to the nines," complete with fancy shoes. I don't think I've really stressed just how determined a woman she was and is—she is an ox, an Aries to boot, after all. Please don't tell her that I think she is probably the most stubborn person that I will ever meet in my lifetime.

Here's my vision of that day, which is partially influenced by my friend Lauren's version of the same story. Lauren had been one of my rocks in this rushing water they call life, and quite ironically one of Granny's as well. Unfortunately this isn't a book about Lauren, but she has heard this waterfall story at least twice, I think. Lauren has told me the same story twice, as well.

So this story is about a day in the 1920s, when "Los Angeles was a dirt road! A dirt road! We smuggled our dog across the border when we moved from Regina . . ."

So imagine, if you will, a sporty Lenore wandering, wondering what the view was like from atop that hill. She manages the climb to the vista, also succeeding in trapping herself on the edge of the cliff. Thankfully she was reported to the authorities, because those fancy shoes weren't going to cut it to reverse the mount.

"THEY SENT A HELICOPTER!" she'd exclaim and look deep into the past. Glazed, she'd gaze into the hardwood floor of the living room and describe the wonder of flying, suspended under the helicopter over a giant waterfall. "IMAGINE THAT! I DIDN'T EVEN KNOW THERE WAS A WATERFALL!" she giggles.

Vivid imagery for seventy-five years, I don't doubt her clarity. Better than digital. The pilot was handsome—I think that was part of the story—well, maybe I'm making that part up. It's a detail that slowly had lost importance or relevance. It is possible to surmise that my granny liked to flirt with handsome gents, and I'll bet that in her tennis skirt, many of her serves were missed by gawking boys.

RANDOM ACTS OF KINDNESS

It isn't always your friends that teach you about virtue and good will. We sometimes are blessed to find that it is strangers who enlighten our spirit with their kindness. Here is such a story, one I've heard many, many times and will do my best to recreate.

Winter is coming.
1958.
First year at Iris Street.
First house on the block.

Lenore is struggling to make it, financially, on her own. She's working for the government, writing contracts. She's been to college and writes shorthand faster than lightning. Until recently, she would still even leave herself notes in shorthand, always holding a secret, I surmise, a reminder perhaps of a wrong done or a clandestine rendezvous. Okay, perhaps the secret romance idea is pushing the buck, but the buck is what this whole story is about. It is about a buck, one dollar a week. It is about a single mother in 1958 with no oil for her furnace and no money in the bank. It is about the $58 between comfort and freezing. It is about a proud woman who wouldn't ask for help.

Most important, it is about a man who owned a furnace oil company, a man who was comfortable, had money in the bank and took the liberty of filling Lenore's tank. Of course, she insisted on payments and if memory serves me correctly, it took her a little over a year, budgeting a dollar a week, to repay this kind stranger. He is a nameless fellow, one who is sure to live on in stories as a gentleman who gave himself to random acts of kindness, and kept Lenore and George warm for their first winter in their new home.

LATE NIGHT THOUGHTS

Granny has rarely, if ever mentioned a movie or television show (apart from tennis matches) in conversation, as a thought or spark of a memory, significant or not. This is just a random late-night flickering of a bigger picture, no pun intended.

Perhaps it's due to her deafness, but whatever its role in society, TV has played little or no role in her life. She was probably too busy for it anyway, her head too full of ideas to be wasting it with idleness. The bottom line is, that medium has left no marks on her.

I am a closet cultural anthropologist—not studying the culture of closets—observing and, generally, keeping my often-shocking opinions to myself. Needless to say, my mind wanders and ponders a lot.

My question: What will members of the TV Generation remember when they're ninety-three?

Will they look into the living room floor and see a waterfall? Or an episode of *Gilligan's Island* or *The Price Is Right*?

LETTING GO

I gave the order to keep her IV out. They had to remove it due to her collapsing veins and the fact that none of the liquid that was going in was coming out. It looked like you could pop her with a sharp stick. Her skin was beginning to ulcerate. She looked like a giant water blister. In order to dry her lungs out they prescribed Scopolamine, somewhat of a last-resort drug, I'm told. "It's really to comfort the family." Really. Really?

Thankfully, my sister had arrived at some point in the madness. We designed a schedule that allowed each of us some downtime and some support. I was so relieved to have her company! Otherwise it's a pretty stark existence going to and from the hospital bed. Granny had dipped into a coma, and without the IV drip she was given a week, maybe two at most.

The Scopolamine was doing its thing: drying out her lungs—and everything else, for that matter. Her tongue had shrunk to a black, leathery stub. We began to spend the days swabbing her lips with those sponges on a lollipop stick. At least it was something to do. We could also clean her teeth with these sponges and gentle mouthwash. Her mouth was all cut up from the seizures. Indeed, the days are long, and the clock on the wall ticks out the seconds just a little too loudly.

Initially, our neighbours stopped in to see how Lenore was doing, but now they stay away. I think they are afraid to see her at the hospital. I'm sure it would break their hearts to see the Matriarch of Iris Street in such a state.

She spent her ninety-third birthday in a coma, a tearful day for family and friends. Everyone is saying goodbye.

I've developed a yoga routine over the bed, holding both her hands. If you squeeze her hand, she squeezes back, or maybe it's a twitch and I'm reading into things. I sing into her hand, she seems to enjoy it.

She still hasn't relieved her bowels.

They switch permanently to a lock for injections because her veins won't take an IV hose. They alternate between the Dilaudid and a sedative: "comfort measures" for end of life. Palliative care. Blah de blah.

All I know is how hard it is to watch and even harder not to. Kristin and I take turns chasing the other home to sleep. The last to leave gets chased by the nursing staff.

A little joy arrives for me when my friend Jody comes on a stopover on her way to the Bahamas. Her excitement is a nice change and uplifting for me. We are just settling in at the house, catching up since our last visit, when the telephone rings. It is Kristin at the hospital. My heart stops.

"Granny's awake! And she's talking!" she sobs. "She says she wants to go home!"

Was she laughing or crying? Am I laughing or crying?

"I gotta go!" she exclaims, "She's trying to escape! Her feet are over the rails now!"

So, once again Granny's will has amazed us all. She wanted to go home. She hadn't eaten or drunk in days, yet she had the strength to verbalize her desire to go home—with her shrivelled tongue. She knew what she wanted and, frankly, I knew that no one would get any rest until she got home—a new path that would lead us to another adventure in the land of caregiving and letting go.

THE NIGHT IS YOUNG

Something's wrong with Granny: she's getting up far too frequently to pee. At least every hour, the motion alarm I have by her bed shocks me out of bed as her feet touch the floor. Not much pee is coming out and it stinks. I remind her to take her walker to the bathroom. She's tipsy—really tired. We both are. I lie on the spare bed while she sits on the toilet and jerk into action when the flush sounds. She always flushes—or always did until the April stroke—and I assist her with pulling up her pajama bottoms. Once again I rest on the spare bed as she carefully washes her hands. I guide her back to bed, tuck her in and say goodnight, at least three times, blow kisses and turn out the light . . . Fall into bed and get up again before I can even determine if I had been asleep.

When the bath lady arrives, I rush off to the clinic and get a urine sample container and ask Granny to fill it. Even at ninety-two, she can squat over the wee cup and fill it with some control. "Didn't spill a drop," she giggles at the achievement.

Indeed, a confirmed bladder infection. The antibiotics arrive that afternoon. It's a sleepy afternoon for both of us, with maybe only eight visits to the toilet that night.

The next morning, Granny wakes with gusto. Her eyes are flashing—I call it "dementia eyes," but I'm sure that's not the medical terminology. Nonetheless, her pupils are dilated. There is an extreme lightness within her eyes, accompanied by a changing shadow, as though a film were flickering with her irises as screens.

It must be February, because we have extra care hours from our care provider. Today our personal care worker is Peggy, a French-Canadian that Granny thinks is "just wonderful and meticulous." Granny still utilizes a large vocabulary of descriptive words with pride.

That morning, we trip. We trip hard, around the house. It's several hours before the bath lady is to arrive, and Granny is acting like she is fifty-five again. Forgetting the walker, she's running around holding the walls for support. I chase after her and attempt to distract her back to the walker, only to do it again and again. She's turning on and off the lights and checking the time.

"IT'S SEVEN-THIRTY? THAT'S TOO EARLY TO GO TO BED!" she declares, like I'm insane to even think that it was bedtime.

I smile and nod and try to get her settled down for breakfast. We have breakfast twice—it is just as good the second time. I'm already exhausted and the day has just begun. Relief fills me when Peggy, the bath lady, arrives and says, "Wow! What's gotten into her?" At least it's not just me. At least I have more than two hours off today . . . having won the care hour lottery.

I call before lunch to check in with Peggy. "Wow!" she says again, "I got to go—she's on the move!"

Not much info—I try again later.

"Wow!" again, "The room's flooding! I gotta go!"

Not enough info—I decide to return home.

Peggy is exhausted. She's had to straighten every picture on all the walls . . . all the cushions are fluffed and arranged like a Martha Stewart magazine. "She sure had me running," she sighs and wishes me luck . . . she'll see us tomorrow at nine.

So I guess it's just me
And Granny
In dementia land
And the night is young.

Donna

Crafty: one of the many words you could use to describe Lenore. I don't know where or when or from whom she learned, but Granny found her calling in creative expression with rug hooking. Not latch-hooking but serious hooking. She even had a sign outside her door that said, "THE HAPPY HOOKER."

Her basement was a studio and a small factory where she would design and prepare hooking projects for her students and herself. Her self-created colour palette was exact and diverse—even the dye company wanted to buy her recipes. With hearing aids on high, she would teach evening art classes to countless students, individuals who still remember her after twenty years of retirement.

Every Friday evening, for about thirty years, Donna would come over to Lenore's. She was probably about thirty and Granny about sixty when their friendship began. Together they were busy little beavers, hovering over hot glue guns, creating any number of toilet paper covers and countless pine cone wreaths for craft shows and presents.

Donna helped Lenore with umpteen projects over the years. Lenore always thought big and was certainly blessed to have Donna's hands and company when completing projects such as the latch-hooking of the Iris Street rugs. They hand-dyed the golden wool for the hall runner, small foot mats and an area rug that filled the living room floor for twenty years. With a wobbly little roller-cutter they kept their arms spinning to cut congruent lengths of yarn. Myself, I remember getting the opportunity to twirl the handle of the "nifty gadget." Granny held it steady for me, as I was using two hands for a one-hand job. I even got to latch a few hooks under Granny's supervision. She'd tighten them down and congratulate me on my fine work.

How ironic it is that we've managed a 360-degree role reversal in my lifetime. Now I hold things steady for her and congratulate her. It still feels good for both of us, I think, to be helping or helped, although I can see it is often difficult for her to even need any help. Kristin said it best: "She's an independent woman who's dependent."

It can't be easy, but it shouldn't be so hard. The only grace of Alzheimer's is that slowly she's forgetting what exactly she used to do before. Before what? Before now, I guess . . . before someone else filled the fridge and paid the bills. She doesn't even ask where the food came from anymore, and I don't think she really wants to know, either.

What fundamentally matters, to both of us, is the moment. The moment in happiness and whatever harmony we can rise to. She's caught in the present, which becomes the past as each breath passes, slipping into oblivion just as quickly.

They say that one of the hardest realities for an elder to face is the loss of the right to drive. It is the ultimate blow to his or her independent ego. Granny managed to live through this shocking change and has let it go. She rarely mentions driving but still keeps her driver's licence in that stone-heavy purse; I carry the purse.

I daresay that it has been far more depressing for her to have to remove those hooked carpets for safety reasons. They were like giant foot-catchers, even to the young and agile. Although I'm sure if anyone fell onto the inch and a half of wool padding, not too many bones would crack on impact.

Those memories are rolled up in the basement now. They flash into her mind from time to time. She certainly remembers the hours spent latching with Donna, and the feel of the rugs under her feet. I'm pretty sure she doesn't remember tripping over them or giving the occupational therapist a run for her money as she tried for nearly a year to convince her to remove them from under foot. I eventually took them all away, a sad day for me, too, before she returned home from respite care with the broken elbow.

I've drifted a little off topic now—forgive me as I steer us back to Donna. There are not a lot of words to describe her dedication to Lenore, and maybe that's enough said. They were like two peas in a pod from two generations. This is a rare connection we all should cultivate with the youth and the elders. It can make you feel good just thinking about it.

I Want to Go Home

I've drifted back to the Queensway Carleton Hospital—well, more like raced—with Jody. Kristin is there, sitting with an upright Granny who's sucking liquid from a sponge. She knows who I am and greets me with warmth. Lets me know that she wants to go home.

I am relieved that she even knows my name. She pretty much always knows who I am except for a few incidents like when those rapist Indians tore through our home one morning. "THEY WERE PRACTICALLY NAKED! IT WAS HORRIBLE!" There were other times that she didn't remember me; or, more correctly, confused me with someone else, usually Evelyn or Donna. Especially Donna—a compliment to me, and I just go along with it to avoid upsetting her. Having just woken up after five (?) days of unconscious slumber, she is a little confused. She wants to go home, as I've already mentioned. She's willing to attempt the journey alone if need be, continually throwing her feet over the bed rails in hopes of reaching a taxi or a miracle. We decide that it's best to hire an overnight attendant to keep her from breaking her neck on the way to the bus and from succumbing to the fear of being alone in a strange place. Emotions run wild on evenings like that, when someone who is accordingly supposed to be dead and is awake. And lucid. And determined.

Once again, I am chased home—with Jody this time, by my sister. I slept really soundly knowing that Barb, a sitter, was with Granny. The hardest thing to do is leave her by herself. Morning comes like a dream, and I'm back in the fourth-floor room, getting the lowdown on Barb's night with Lenore: a lot of mouth-swabbing and countless escape attempts. They are both exhausted, but not too tired to keep from trying to go home. Her arms freeze-lock on the rails and she wiggles her feet to the end of the bed where there's a small space for feet between the rail and the foot of the bed. She must have felt a small sense of freedom to have even just her toes free from the confinement of the bed. It takes two people to get her properly back into bed. This makes her very agitated, so they sedate her. That is how our day goes.

It seems her only true pain is in her belly; granted, she still hasn't had a shit—so they give her more Dilaudid for pain, which consequently constipates her even more.

I decide to take her home. It's hard to keep her settled; if I haven't mentioned, she wants to go home. A few details must be worked out first, of course, so the waiting game starts with the goal to be back at home. Home is where the heart is.

She qualifies for private nursing—yee hoo!—it's cheaper to send a nurse than keep her in hospital. Well, that is, she qualified for nursing until she took a sip of water. It was the sip that changed her status. If she drinks water, she won't be dead in a week . . . so she no longer qualifies for anything except drop-in nursing and three months with a free hospital bed. Okay. Whatever. All we need is a doctor now, due to the fact that her GP has refused to treat her in her current condition.

We wait in vain for several days for a palliative care practitioner. We eventually give up and take her home anyway. She's losing it in that room, and frankly so am I. Her will to go home is unbreakable. Kristin has to return to work, too, and I know I can't handle the hospital alone for any more time.

The hospital bed arrived at four p.m. and Granny at five-fifteen p.m. I've converted the living room into a hospital.

She is content.

Albeit, a little confused to be sleeping where the dining room table should be, but nonetheless she is content.

She doesn't try to escape—she is at peace to be at home.

Yes, we have no doctor.

Yes, we have a bunch of wonderful ladies hovering. "My angels," Granny declares.

And my angels, too.

THE NIGHT IS STILL YOUNG

I really couldn't understand the flooding in the living room comment. Peggy can't understand what is wrong with the TV. When I arrive home she's puzzling over the unplugged television, trying to fix it. The show that's on is disturbing Granny. "WHY WOULD THEY SHOW SUCH HORRIBLE THINGS ON TELEVISION?"

She's very agitated with the show that's playing from the unplugged machine. Peggy is exhausted. I realize that it's the reflecting light that has her hot and bothered, so I cover the screen with a large painting, a simple solution to this perplexing problem. We wave goodbye to Peggy, and I catch up on the new wave of happenings in our little world.

The flooding is hard to control. Water is pooling into the living room in all directions. An absolutely horrified Granny is screeching, "THE WATER WILL MARK THE FLOORS! I'D BETTER MOP IT UP!"

I'll tell you, even if you already know, that the last thing a ninety-two-year-old should be doing is bending over with a rag, one hand on a walker—with the brakes off—to mop the floor. I take over the chore of eradicating the lake forming in the house. She is inspecting, pointing and screaming, "WATER! WATER! EVERYWHERE!"

We spend about three hours mopping and mopping invisible water into an empty bucket. Just as I finish one side of the room, the waterfall flows in on the other side. My arms were getting tired—let alone my mind. I am chasing her around the house, turning off the taps she's turned on, reverently mopping the aggravating waters that are plaguing our home. Where is all the water coming from? Where are all the bugs from?

Indeed, there are bugs all over the place; not slowed by the flooding floors, they are scuttling up the walls and all over the ceiling. Crawling over just about everything.

I don't really know what to do. I'm trying to convince her to go to bed and close her eyes, otherwise I, myself, might start seeing things. Her eyes are darting. I turn down the lights to stop the reflections on the floors and possibly calm the bugs down, grasping—that's me—grasping at straws—praying that this high action day will knock her out for the night. Maybe she won't need to pee eight times tonight.

With lots of ifs and maybes, I eventually get her changed and tucked into bed. A sigh starts my night. A sigh and a selfish prayer, one that was getting to be a common wish: please let me sleep tonight. Please.

Laura and Anna

They say that there are no coincidences in life. Having two little girls move in across the street was certainly a fateful circumstance for Lenore, Anna, and Laura. Growing up, we lived two hours away, and I do recall a hint of jealousy on my part as a child knowing that pretty much every day, these two beautiful girls got to sit on my Granny's swing, eating her cookies and listening to her read aloud *The Little House on the Prairie.*

She was "The Swinging Granny" by this point in time, retiring the old "Happy Hooker" sign with this coming of age.

I'm positive that the benefits of the friendship will live on in the girls for their lifetime, as they are sure to have young ladies popping over when they are seventy-five, perhaps to reread the same novels as they sip cold drinks and munch on shortbread.

It wasn't until I moved to Ottawa to live with Granny that I got the pleasure of getting to know them. Laura, at this time, was off in Taiwan but her letters arrived regularly with photos and stories for Granny. As my life unfolds in Ottawa, it is Anna that is Granny's most dedicated visitor, and mine, too, for that matter. She checks in on us and helps me to pacify Granny's desire for eating out. Together we guide her over ice and snow, into restaurants and cafés where we are doomed to stick in till we stick out.

Anna is one of the few visitors who really takes the time to write and interact with her. She has a fabulous sense of humour, an asset for both of us, especially on the tumultuous evening we spent together beside the hospital bed in the living room. I think it was the evening that the Indians raided, raped, and pillaged Iris Street—Granny was still in another dimension. Her bed was soiled with the blood of a miscarriage. Hearts in hand, we tried our best to comfort her through this tragedy.

For Lenore, eleven pregnancies stopped short and broke her heart. George was the blessed one that made it to term and will always be the apple of her eye.

I was beginning to realize that the drugs weren't doing much good at all, for any of us. I had been sent home from the Queensway Carleton with a quick how-to and a bag of heavy drugs. Being family, I could administer the needles, legally, that is. The night-shift ladies would wake me every few hours to dose her up, and I would help to roll her over and prop her up with every pillow in the house.

The sedative was making her agitated and the Dilaudid had her trapped in a past of unresolved reminiscences. After consulting the visiting nurse (we still had no doctor), we decided to wean her off the drugs.

My sister had left at this point, and the house was a full-blown hospital. Every morning after her sponge bath, we rolled the bed to the window so she could see the birds and traffic. I felt as though I hadn't a moment to myself. Uncertainty has hooked itself into our lives and warped the present into a slow-moving liquid. Luckily, I haven't the time to consider the future. Head to the grindstone, I pushed myself on through Granny's recovery.

And recovery was what it was. The visiting nurse said it best: "Holy Crap! What are you feeding her?" A compliment regarding the miraculous advances Granny was making.

I am pretty sure that had we left her at the hospital, she probably would have taken the one-way ticket to the afterlife. In her own domain, however, surrounded by the familiar, she was able to find the peace to heal. She quickly regained words, skills, and mobility. The biggest change for her was the wheelchair—she doesn't want to use the walker anymore.

Selfishly, I appreciate the rails on the hospital bed, as they eliminate the late-night adventures. She hates the rails but is learning to accept them. I bet my average sleep time has doubled. How did I manage before?

They do say that what doesn't kill you will make you stronger.

A STRONG, INDEPENDENT WOMAN

Today, I told Granny that she started the women's revolution. She agreed and smiled.

I didn't have to explain my reasoning; she understood completely. We had a cup of tea and sat in silence, a comfortable silence. It is important to share her silence—her silent world.

NOT A FUNNY BONE

It's not that I can't believe how mixed-up this time has become in my mind. I just found an old note of incidents and am shocked at myself. It wasn't the antibiotics for a bladder infection that started Granny's spin around dementia land, with the floods and the bugs. The bladder infection did occur, but looking back I realize that happened just after she returned home from respite care, where she spent almost six weeks in a wet diaper. We did get up countless times a night to pee during the infection, but she didn't go off the deep end that time she took antibiotics. So please excuse the confusion.

They say that caregivers are often forgetful. It is a sign of stress. The story should have gone something like this:

Granny's broken elbow (now apparently fixed) was driving us crazy. She was in agony most of the time. It was red as a tomato and hot enough to fry an egg on. That's why she was on antibiotics. One of the many falls she had in respite care had resulted in a superficial skin infection . . . right on top of the broken bones. It was assumed that the infection was still present under the surface, festering. The fall also pushed those newly set bones all askew, dislodging a wire that was holding the whole mess together. Instead of keeping it all in place, the wire was rattling around in there, chopping up her tissue with its sharp and twisted ends. My notes remind me now that it wasn't peeing that primarily kept us up those nights, but the agony in her funny bone and the ringing in her ears. The hallucinations didn't help, either. They never do.

It's the flooding night and I'm so relieved to be lying down, when the talking starts. By now, I'm used to her sleep-talking, jibberish, mind you, and tonight she is making sense, complete sentences. Her motion alarm gets me up and back into the swing of the evening.

She's up and talking with unseen bodies—unseen to me but tangible to her. The people in her room do not include her husband; he would arrive later, in the wee hours of the morning.

She's angry with these folks, though, and is screaming, "LEAVE ME ALONE! YOU'LL HAVE TO LEAVE!" She escorts them to the door, and I convince them never to come back. Then I convince Granny that they won't be coming back and get her settled into bed. Our night goes sort of like that—one scene after the other. I am busy chasing the ghosts from our presence and calming Granny down. In a moment of quiet, I even called Telehealth, who advised me to call an ambulance. "They'll sedate her and strap her down," the nurse reassures me. Lovely. I bear down and decide to make it on my own until morning. I've given up trying to sleep. Deprivation is like that. Eventually it's easier to stay awake than to sleep. Getting back up is way too hard, anyway.

All thoughts of slumber aside, we are too busy shopping to nod off anyway. Granny's bargaining with salesmen: "FIVE DOLLARS? WOW! PACK IT UP! I'LL TAKE IT!" and, "67.89? HMMMM. THAT'S A LITTLE TOO DEAR FOR MY BLOOD. I'LL HAVE TO THINK ABOUT IT . . ." hinting that a deal could be made, if the price were right.

So much happened that night that it is a blur. I know that we both laughed and cried as the worlds opened before us. It is breakfast time before we know it. I'm too weary to give her the morning dose of antibiotics, but the Telehealth nurse had said, "No one reacts to those drugs in such a peculiar manner." Ten minutes after the pill is down the hatch, I'm amazed to watch her upper lip start to swell. I contact her GP, who suggests stopping the drugs and giving her Benedril™. The bath lady isn't due for a while yet, so I telephone a neighbour to come and sit with Granny while I zip to the drugstore. Thankfully, the antihistamine works, and the swelling slowly disappears from her lips and face.

It's been a long, long day, two days long with long nights connecting them. When I put Granny to bed, she sleeps the night away, most of the next day and the next night, too, just enough time for both of us to feel sane again.

Part of her is extremely at peace—not just an exhausted calm, either. Perhaps all those visits to the past have released some of the emotional baggage she has been lugging around.

After a few very slow-moving days, I am ready to take a crack at a new antibiotic. She has a similar reaction, only quicker this time, so our hands are tied with what to do. Without many options we end up back at the Civic Hospital after another long night of screaming pain in the arm. The funny bone that never was—funny, that is.

STILL NOT A FUNNY BONE

Cheryl came almost immediately after I phoned for help. It was the first time I was smart enough to phone for help; I'd learned the hard way what standing alone too long can do to my spirit. We were in emergency for eight hours before Cheryl arrived and were lucky to have a concerned intern who really listened to our crazy story. Previous tests done on her elbow showed only a superficial infection, but that day they discovered a deeper infection brewing in the elbow. Cheryl stayed with Granny while she awaited a room and I headed home to catch some sleep. Bone scans and other tests would commence the following day. The hospital would monitor her carefully for allergic reactions to the antibiotics.

It was the break in that funny bone that had ended her independence four months prior to this visit to the Civic. It was that October phone call that changed my life. It was surely the morphine that kicked her Alzheimer's into gear. A social worker told me that she would never walk again and she would have to go into a home.

For me, it was an eye-opening, heartbreaking time, hitting like a tidal wave in our lives. My mother came from Calgary to keep me floating along this path of Power of Attorney for Personal Care, the alternative decision maker, deciding what Granny would want if she could decide for herself. We surveyed the possible placement opportunities and brought home with us images of vacant eyes or worse still, those sad and pleading puppy eyes that haven't the words or perhaps the will to describe their loss of control of reality, humility, and pride, or the power to change it.

The where am I of who I was?
Was I?
Where did everybody go?

GUILTY CONSCIENCE GETS ME GOOD

I'll tell you that putting Granny in a home, even in a temporary placement, was the hardest thing that I have ever done. Granted, at first she thought it was a hospital; but even with Alzheimer's and on megadoses of Tylenol 3™, one can't overlook reality for too long. I was still working and commuting for my days off to spend with Granny in her new home.

I'd spend the day there trying to get her to eat—she'd decided to starve rather then spend too much more time there. I can't blame her. Perhaps if she hadn't been deaf she could have gotten into some activities or even communicated with some of the individuals on her floor. Contracting the flu probably didn't encourage her to stay. Falling probably wasn't on the plus side, either.

I'd say I was having a nervous breakdown of sorts. Guilt had me in its clutches, and I was useless at making even simple decisions, let alone deciding where to place Granny permanently for her last days. She'd tell me over and over,

"I wish I were dead, Heather."

Again and again.

Wearing me down with each minute of every visit.

"I want to go home, Heather"

I remember waking up with chapped eyelids that only days of crying can cause. It was that day that I decided to step up to bat for Granny and my mood finally lifted. It was that day when a profound and historic moment of clarity moved me from the bowels of uncertainty and gave me the strength to go ahead with my plan to move in with Granny and care for her. I'd always known inside myself, deep inside, that I would be caring for my wonderful Granny. I hadn't envisioned diapers and temper tantrums, but I did have a hint of my fate for years leading up to that autumn day, when my heart changed my life.

Joy filled me as I made plans to bring Granny home.

BRING GRANNY HOME!

That night, the gods and goddesses thanked me for my sacrifice. They gave me a gift, a sign, as the northern skies opened up and danced the night away with me. I sat in peace, spellbound, to watch the aurora borealis define the heavens with their mystical beauty.

For me, it was an affirmation that the right path had fallen at my feet, one where Granny and I would share, rough or smooth, a road filled with love that could conquer the adversity of growing up, growing old, and growing together.

HEAVEN CAN WAIT

Even through all her pain, suffering and confusion, a bouquet of daisies causes her to proclaim wholeheartedly, "HEAVEN CAN WAIT!" She says it nearly every day about something. Mostly about birds, sunsets, fancy desserts, long car rides, and walks in the wheelchair down the bike trail by the creek. "HEAVEN CAN WAIT!" is a strong statement, at ninety-three or at twenty-three, and she says it with every ounce of her being, over and over again.

She is incredibly thankful for everything. Combined with her forgetfulness, she can thank me—thank anyone—all day for the little things that are done for her. The simplest things please her and she wants nothing more than to make sure that she remembers to thank people, even if she overdoes it.

We are lucky she hasn't lost her social graces, like many Alzheimer's patients. Her dignity will be the last thing to go, I'm sure, in this battle she is fighting to remain wholly and purely Lenore. Since the big stroke and all the drugs, many little things have slipped from her routine and personality. These details are all fundamentally unimportant in the greater scheme of things. I mean, if I have to suggest with a hand gesture that somebody stand up to get on the toilet, so be it—it really doesn't take too much more energy on my part. The most important thing is to let her do what she can do, even if it takes longer to complete; she still gets joy from finishing a small chore. Quite honestly, she gets more enjoyment out of simple chores than anyone I've ever known. Which I assume is the reason that heaven can wait if a butterfly flits by while we're on the swing.

I try to keep positive, even though things are slipping. Some days it's two steps back, but then there are two-step-forward days to balance it all out. The only virtue I can grasp from this disease is that the little things really matter—they make or break the day for us. Like kisses. Lots of kisses for Granny means a good day. It's an easy requirement to fill, for me, anyway, and I can keep her happy just by blowing a kiss across the room. Perhaps we all need to keep an open heart for the wee things in life, take notice and the time to appreciate them. In the end, these things, great but small, are all that matter enough to make heaven wait.

RECOVERY

I think that Betty and Audrey are here with Granny and me. We're still recovering from the stroke, so it is a tag-team job. Two people need to be here most of the time to keep moving her to avoid bedsores and just to keep things rolling along.

Betty has been coming every second weekend since January to provide fifty hours of much-needed respite. It is the perfect set-up, partly because she's totally thorough, competent, and kind, and partly because she lets me stay at her beautiful house on the lake. I try not to do anything but things for me: do yoga, play music, swim, ski, visit friends, see my dog, eat spicy food, and sleep. Sleeping is the most important thing. One weekend I slept for twenty-seven hours. I guess I was tired or something.

Betty does more than just stay with Granny. She has been a main support outlet for me. She's listened to me more times than I can count: when I am occasionally freaking out and when I am unsure, which is often. She isn't afraid of any possible situations that can and might occur.

When I return home on Sunday afternoons, she has the house looking great. Cleaning has been a problem for me at Granny's, not the act of cleaning but the not getting caught part. I haven't tried in a while, but if Granny sees me vacuuming she shrieks louder than the Kenmore, "DON'T DO THAT, HEATHER! YOU'RE MY GUEST! I'LL DO IT! LET ME DO IT!" Maybe now from the wheelchair she won't attempt to take the vacuum from me, or even want to try. Most likely, seeing me vacuum reminds her of one terrible thought: that she's unable to do it anymore—and that she's not quite sure of that—and what's more, that she's not willing to admit it.

So we're gathered around the hospital bed—Audrey, and Betty, and myself. I'm beyond exhausted. My plan is to stay with the ladies for twenty-four hours and show them our new routine: charts to keep track of what goes in and what goes out, how to roll her, bathing and oral hygiene, massaging to keep her skin from breaking down, medicine for pain relief, pureeing food, and any number of other details it takes to run a one-person hospital. Someone always sleeps on the couch beside her. She is often scared in the night and thirsty. Maybe she'll even eat a few bites of food at midnight. There is a flow to providing this kind of care and I had no reservations leaving Granny in their care. They are both competent and confident women.

Granny was obviously recovering, marked by her first bowel movement in seventeen days—the kind of thing that made your eyes water—a sure sign that things were starting to work again.

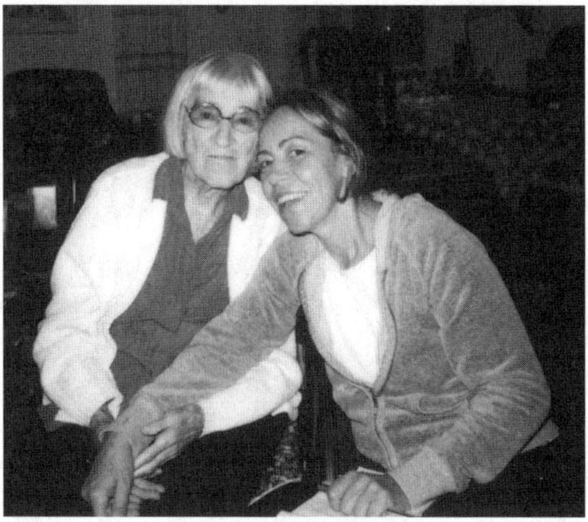

Lenore and Betty

Anyway, there we are, with Granny relatively lucid and in the present moment, a wonderful change to see. She doesn't understand why the ladies are there, and she certainly doesn't understand the seriousness of her condition. She is the centre of attention, though, and she captivates with everything she says, even if it doesn't make much sense.

This is what she said, almost word for word, I think.

"HEATHER." Wow. She knows my name. I'm tickled pink. I have a selfish fear that one day she won't recognize me.

"HEATHER, YOU SHOULD WRITE A BOOK OF MY LIFE:
A FARMER PLANTED A SEED
I PLANTED THE TREE
THE END."

GRANNY'S MAPLE TREE

There's not a lot you can say after a story like that. Maybe a little background is good. It is a beautiful maple tree that stands in her front yard—the nicest on the block. I can truly say to people, "It's the house with the big tree," and I do say that because you can't see the house number in the summer for all the leaves. The branches pull at your sweater when you get in or out of your car. She cried once (sobbing), when my dad clipped the eye-level branches. She'd rather have someone go blind than have that tree snipped or snapped—really; no joking about that tree.

She loves her tree.

She planted the tree.

If you had met her a few months ago, she'd have told you that she planted it in 1959.

She still knows that she planted that beautiful tree but really doesn't care when she planted it. The when part really doesn't matter anymore and that's an important fact all on its own. Slowly the when of things doesn't matter in the big scheme.

It is also important to note that in those few words about her life she never mentioned her thirty-five years in a government job, or years of teaching, or even having a family, winning tennis championships, losing her best friend, her hearing, and eleven unborn children. The most important thing at that moment and probably many moments in her life was the tree she planted her first year free from abuse, in front of her own home.

She watched that tree grow into its majestic pose, and the tree got to see her grow into hers as well. When Granny passes on, that tree might just want to fall over with her.

And it probably will.

HELP IS CLOSE TO HOME

If I wasn't struggling before the April stroke, then I don't know what I was doing after it. In many respects I was a whole lot wiser, not only in terms of medical know-how and clinical how-to but on a deeper level of knowing and understanding life. Death is a big part of life for a small part of the time; for the living as well as for those passing on, I suppose. It happens to everyone who lives—dying, that is, even to those who strive to be saved in glass jars for the future. I was lucky enough to be very close to my granny all my life and know her wishes in regards to her death. She always told me that she didn't want to make anyone sad and that she should be shipped directly to the university where they could study her ears and maybe they could save someone from living in a silent world like she did. She's so very thoughtful and direct. She also told me that she paid for her funeral, long, long ago, probably to the detriment of the funeral home, which must have sorely undercharged her. Who'd've foreseen that she'd live this long? I'm sure it would thrill her to know just how much money she is saving, even from the grave.

She also verbalized her desire to die naturally. No machines, etcetera. Her Power of Attorney for Personal Care spells it out clear as day: *Let me go if it's time. Only keep me comfortable and otherwise let me be*. That's obviously not how the document was written, but close enough.

Having to tell the doctors to stop—STOP!—was a terribly hard thing for me to do, even if I knew that was what she wanted. It took a really long walk and a lot of tears. Am I ready to say goodbye? Isn't that the most selfish question I can ask myself? Like my loss is more important than her loss, being the agony of living on and on, perhaps unable to communicate or move.

Thankfully for me, Granny's body didn't want the IV, and removal of it was a necessity. I did, however, request that they leave it out and let her pass on without lingering for months in a bloated coma. I made that decision after a long walk, like I said, after a hard day at the hospital, a day when after for so long being in a coma, Granny opened her eyes. They were white, completely white. There was a hint of grey where her pupils should have been but the rest was white. I couldn't believe my eyes—her eyes. I'd hoped for her to see me, for the comfort of both of us, when and if she ever awoke again. She couldn't see my hand flap in front of her. She couldn't see. She knew she couldn't see, too, and made a bunch of horrifying sounds with her shrivelled stub of a tongue. She blinked hard and moaned and wailed. I think then she gave up. I really can't imagine what would have gone through her mind in those minutes; hopefully she couldn't grasp the ramifications of being deaf and blind in the few waking moments.

If not, then why the tears she shed?

What she didn't grasp, I surely did. I was and am at a loss for words to describe my feelings that day. I had to 'fess up that holding onto her for me was not what this was about. It really doesn't matter what anyone says, right or wrong, telling the hospital to let someone die is hard all around, even if you know what is right. Prolonging life is sometimes prolonging suffering. In retrospect, the decision came easier to me than when I had to place her into a "home." It's a little more final—death, that is, but choosing someone's life course was, in reality, a far more challenging task than allowing her to die.

To make a long story draw to a close, letting Granny choose her own path was the best road to take. She chose to live. She opened her eyes for a few more blind attempts, and a few days later her eyes cleared up and she could see again. No one ever ascertained what happened to cause her eyes to glaze over, but things happen, and they happen for reasons we may never ever know. We must always have faith in that fact. We may never know even the question, but the answers will be clear when the time is right. I can and must have patience for that.

Which brings me to the point of this whole interlude. Anna had been coming pretty much every evening to be with us. Thank you. Thank you. I told the staff she was a granddaughter and she truly is, of the heart, which is all that matters in times like these. She told Laura of Granny's imminent death, and Laura flew home from Taiwan. This is not a trip to the corner store. When she arrived,

Granny was already home and beginning to form sentences again. I know that Granny is well-loved by these girls, beyond love that any amount of family could give. I begged her not to return to Taiwan and to work for us over the summer. "I need help," I pleaded.

That's how I got to be sane for the summer and how Laura got a crash course in personal care. She has been an asset to our home and lives. Granny loves her and they groove together. It's important for Granny that Laura is a constant in her life; they are comfortable together, at home with each other. It makes it easy for me to come and go without training a new stranger in the routines and rhythms of our lives every time I go out dancing or to a dentist appointment. I'm a little worried about the fall, when university starts for Laura. I daresay that I'm now spoiled by my time off and hope I can manage without as much freedom. I'm sure I'll be fine. I'll have faith that everything will work out for the best. For everyone.

TISSUES, TISSUES, EVERYWHERE

I have to laugh—just about every night I have to laugh at the quantity of Kleenex that my granny can stash hither and thither on her person. Kleenex must be a luxury if you were born in 1912, a luxury that my granny luxuriates with. She gives me one Kleenex with every meal, maybe two if she's forgotten the first. That's how her day goes, one forgotten Kleenex after another, tucked up sleeves, in pockets of pants, sweaters, and even under the straps of her brassiere.

At night, it's like a snowstorm in the washroom as they appear and tumble to the floor, one after another. Needless to say, even after a good shaking, I miss many a tissue— at least one Kleenex per wash, each load sprinkled with tiny balls of paper, creating another activity for Granny as she folds the laundry and compulsively picks the pieces off. That's what those fabric softeners are for, they gather up the Kleenex, and the filter is full of them. There are just enough Kleenex balls left to warrant being an activity for her. She loves to fold the laundry. She beams when I bring it to her. She glows when I take the folded laundry away.

I will tell you a little secret, one I'm sure you can keep under your hat . . .

If Granny is caught in a cycle of thought, which happens as often as she forgets, I sometimes create a little laundry folding for her. Socks are the best, as they take a little thought to organize and coordinate. I talked to an Alzheimer's counsellor one day and admitted that I periodically do this make-work project of unfolding various articles and messing them up for her! "Brilliant!" she says, "I'll suggest that to other caregivers!"

And here I thought that I was being cruel in some way, although the outcome is generally the same: Granny feels useful and proud. I praise her and kiss her. The thing that was upsetting her is forgotten in the matched-up socks and perfectly folded facecloths.

It's also funny to note that if only half of a set of pajamas is in the load, she doesn't know what to do with it. Normally she would fold and match the items, but when there is only one of them, she is at a loss and puts the unfolded piece aside. I make it disappear and all is well.

FARIEL

I've mentioned Fariel earlier on, perhaps not by name, but she is our regular "bath lady." That's what Granny calls her, and anyone who comes to help her bathe and dress.

Fariel comes to Iris Street Central every morning at nine o'clock, except lately she has been taking Friday mornings off for herself. Together we go to wake Granny, if she's still snoozing, which I like because then I have at least an hour or two to myself before our day begins. My morning time is incredibly important to me. I do a copious amount of things during this Granny-free time. Of course, I have the baby monitor strapped on in case she wakens and needs me. I set up for the day, mentally preparing for nurses, doctors, and visitors, make grocery lists, do housework, do yoga, pay bills, sing a song or two on the guitar, and even dance about the kitchen with some music on, low enough, of course, to hear her little brass bell tinkle if she needs me. Or we may have had a bad night and I might even still be asleep when the buzzer rings and Fariel is at the front door with a smile.

She works for an agency that is hired by our community care centre to provide the maximum allotted personal care for Ontario residents: fifteen hours a week. This is a steadfast rule, as I discovered when I requested more help; a rule governed by the Ministry of Health and Long Term Care. There is a lot of wind blowing that sail. What direction it is blowing, is beyond me; if this were a political novel I'd start ranting now, but fortunately this is a book about caring, and I can spare you the agony of all my words. I can spare myself, as well, from wasting my wind in expressing my frustration. Technically, Granny should be in a nursing home, according to the system available to us. Our society is built for that, putting our elders in nursing homes, that is. If this were an infrastructure debate, I would still be ranting, and you'd be begging for someone, anyone, to please shut this girl up. Point taken; no more comments.

So, the agency sends a personal care worker to our home every day. We are blessed with Fariel, who is dedicated to Lenore beyond the call of duty. She brings roses from her garden and mangoes to share. When she first arrived on the scene, she graciously ate a second breakfast, just to get Granny to eat. Now she brings her breakfast with her, a must in getting Granny to partake in the most important meal of the day.

That's how Granny's day starts: Fariel and I appearing in her bedroom with good morning kisses, eye drops, choosing an outfit, and off to the bathroom they go. I disappear for my two hours free of baby monitors and having to write notes. I walk, bike, go for groceries, go to the library, perhaps visit a friend, or my favourite—going to a green-space to space out. Having a shower is also a luxury while someone is there to monitor Granny's actions.

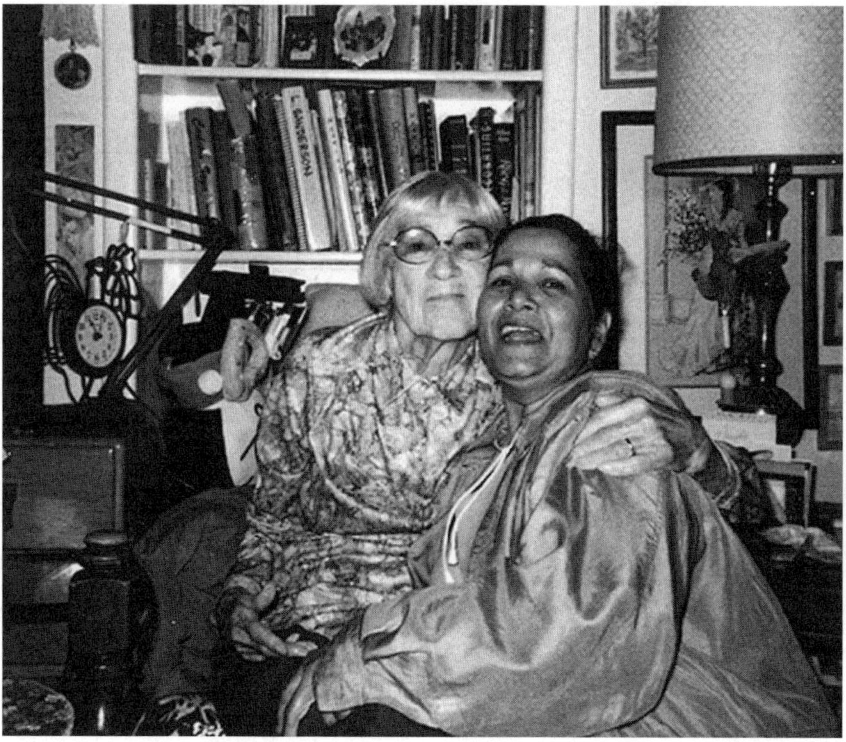

Lenore and Fariel

Meanwhile, under the maple tree, Fariel and Granny have had a bath, got dressed, put on jewellery, had breakfast, done the dishes, and gone to relax in the living room. They sit and chat about flowers and birds until Granny dozes off; she is comfortable enough with Fariel to allow herself the pleasure of a morning snooze. Fariel then changes the bed, cleans the bathroom, tidies the kitchen, prepares the laundry, fills out her "chores done" list and her time slip. By then, I've returned home and we all sit together until eleven o'clock when Granny and I wave Fariel goodbye.

It is a busy two hours for the bath lady, especially when you have to write everything down in conversation. Fariel follows the rules—she works for an agency after all—but she also works from the heart and soul. As I've already said, Granny is blessed by her help and company. I'm sure there is a higher calling bonding these two. For one thing, Granny isn't racist anymore. She used to say things like, "Black people are dirty." That was her upbringing and I don't blame her for her opinions but commend her for her ability to change, evolve, and accept, even grow to love this wonderful woman who has dedicated every morning of the past long while to starting the day right, with one bite for every bite at Lenore's kitchen table.

AFTER A FEW CORONAS AND ANOTHER LONG DAY

Sometimes I wonder if I am crazy to be doing this.
I don't think so, though.
Sometimes I know that something extraordinary is taking place.
But only slowly taking form.
I know it is something about patience.
I know it is everything about love.
Sometimes I dare to think about the future.
I don't want to tease myself with plans.
I don't know where we're going.
I don't know where I'm going, either.
It seems to me that those who do "know" are pretty fucked-up anyway.
It is about living in the moment.
It is about giving without wanting anything in return.
I am realizing lessons daily.
They are, by nature, quiet lessons.
They are slow and lingering.
They are mine.
Mine to share.
Mine to keep.
Mine to cherish.

And cherish I shall do.

JAGGED PERCEPTION

It's my turn for jagged perception, now. I'm realizing just how jagged this book must seem; not only am I talking both in the past and the present but I'm talking in the present in the past. I have yet to make the present the past—that happens pretty quickly and naturally all on its own.

If I'm talking in the present, are you there too? If you are thinking, then it must be working.

I always remember, or half-remember, something I read written on a wall somewhere in the deep woods near Killaloe, the Elephant Men wailing another rendition of "Knockin' on Heaven's Door" in the background. I can't accredit the author because he/she is unknown to me, but I do know whose hands painted these words on the wall:

"I'm not sure you really understand that what you think I thought I said is not really what I meant."

It went something like that, anyway, and it sort of hits the nail on the head.

FINDING HELP

I have gone, to date, to one Alzheimer's support group meeting. It was, for me, an affirmation that I was doing things well, for me and for Granny. It was February and we had won the "extra care hours lottery"—100 extra hours of personal care services; 100 extra hours of freedom. Quite honestly, I wouldn't have gone to the meeting otherwise, due to the expense of hiring a sitter.

Some caregivers don't realize that they need time off for themselves; luckily I have a strong sense of self and figured that out all on my own. That is not my problem; finding the help is the problem. At least I know that I need help: the first step to keeping sane in this realm.

According to the Alzheimer's Society, I am the youngest caregiver in the Ottawa region that they know of. However, if there are other young caregivers like me out there they probably don't have time to be popping into support group meetings either and will probably remain unknown to societies everywhere. They may even be slipping through the cracks.

I was thirty when I went to that meeting, grouped with spouses and children of Alzheimer's victims. One woman that was present was dedicated to a fault to her ailing mother and finally had to give in to long-term care placement when she herself had fallen ill. She was still recovering from that journey with her mother. I'm really not supposed to talk about the meeting, all is confidential; so I will tell you what I learned in those few hours.

The one fact that can hit a caregiver hard between the eyes is that thirty percent of Alzheimer's caregivers die before their patient. Doing the math, I calculate that if Granny lives to be 100, I have a thirty percent chance of dropping dead before I'm forty. That's one to gnaw on. I'm pretty certain that the statistics are based on an older caregiver average age and take it with a grain or two of salt.

Why do they drop dead? It must be related to stress, I surmise. I have to wonder about the medical costs for treating stress-related disorders in caregivers? I'm positive this expense is far greater than a provision made for **respite**, which would also create jobs and alleviate the strain on long-term care facilities for both permanent and respite care placement.

Most importantly, I learned that I am not alone in the grief I feel, the sadness that lingers with losing some parts of Granny that I truly loved and miss. I hope that these memories remain strong for me and aren't jaded, with her sometimes twatty behaviour and these circumstances that keep arising but are beyond our control and imagination.

If you're thinking about jumping into the care boat, the only advice I can give you is this: You can't be prepared for everything (or anything, for that matter). But be prepared anyway. A doctor friend of mine told me, "Well, Deedee [that is my common name, a nickname that Granny doesn't use], expect the unexpected. That's all you can do." All in all, it's very broad and vague advice, but words of wisdom are never clear as day. It has been the best advice I have gotten on this journey.

There are no rules here, just be agile and flexible. Look after yourself first, even when you're more concerned about your partner. The bottom line is happiness—that of the patient *and* the caregiver. I always keep in mind that everything could be over in a flash or go on and on and on. The only way to keep my head up in this stream is to remind myself that every day is a gift, for myself and for Granny. It is a present to hold onto and a presence to let go of all at once.

Looking at the bigger picture, all our lives are temporary and fragile. Accepting death, of loved ones and ourselves, makes living for the moment the only path to follow. This is probably the fundamental lesson in end-of-life care, a bit of wisdom to engage throughout life, not just when the end is imminent.

Here's to the now; it's already past and we have another now to cherish. All in a day in the life. Heaven can wait.

DANCING FOOL, DANCING

Over the winter, I would take an evening off on during the week before Betty would come. Initially, I would come home after a night of dancing, but only too soon did I realize that coming home at two a.m. and getting up repeatedly until the bath lady arrived really didn't leave me in any shape to cope, or even hope to get through the next day. It was almost cheaper to hire an overnight sitter anyway, so I eventually started to crash on a friend's couch and go home to meet the bath lady for an eleven o'clock shift change. Back then I was really concerned with the financial cost of my going out, an anxiety I have been forced to let go of. I now realize that the cost of freedom has no bounds. Okay, to a point—I try not to abuse it, but I also don't beat myself up if that money gets spent and I can have a good time.

I love the island music, African rhythms—well, I love all music, but can really shake it down to funky grooves and reggae. As luck would have it, there is a reggae night in Ottawa; it is a jam, so a variety of colourful musicians keep the music flowing. The crowd is far from mainstream, no ties or suits here—lots of tie-dye and hip-huggers fill the dance floor. I will say quite honestly that without this release, I would have given up . . . given up what? Hmmm. A small part of myself, I guess, the small part that is the spark behind the flame.

I say "release" in the highest sense of the word, equivalent to an epiphany or a spiritual healing. It happened to me twice, once when I was alone, and once with my two girlfriends, both times to the same song. If you're not familiar with Bob Marley, you should go out and buy any of his albums, the older the better, and let his words sink under your skin. That's what happened to me; the music got into me . . . under me . . . through me as I danced. I was smiling, I was laughing, and then the tears started. I was flowing like a waterfall, laughing and crying and dancing—and I didn't care who saw my emotions let go on the dance floor. I hugged myself as they sang, "One good thing about music, when it hits you feel no pain . . ." I'd write out all the words for this song, but if you don't know it, it is reason enough to purchase the album.

Needless to say, on those two instances, I went home about a thousand pounds lighter, in weight and in shade, my spark renewed. We all have triggers within that can start the healing process; thankfully my liberation involves music and dancing, a simple key to releasing stagnant and often harrowing energies. So I will be a dancing fool, for the rest of my life. You'll see me in fields and dreams, letting the music soothe my soul, a passive way to revive and awaken, pure and simple.

MRS. IRIS STREET

There is a single dad across the street who has stopped in a few times to see how Granny was, after late-night paramedic visits. He asked me how Mrs. Iris Street was. That's what his family calls her—Mrs. Iris Street. Now he knows that she is Mrs. Sanderson, but it brings a smile to my face to think of Mrs. Iris Street, the first person to live on Iris Street, in the first house built there. Forty-seven years have passed for her under the tree she planted.

She was very lucid yesterday and told me, "I MOVED HERE IN THE WINTER. THERE WAS NOTHING ACROSS THE STREET. NOTHING! AND IN THE SPRING, BOY, DID I GET THE SHOCK OF MY LIFE! WHEN THE SNOW MELTED THE ROAD WAS DIRT! I STILL CAN'T BELIEVE IT! DIRT!"

I said, "Wow, you've seen a lot of changes in those forty-seven years."

"Forty-seven YEARS?" eyes wide. "TIME SURE FLIES!" she laughed. Mrs. Iris Street sighed and peered out into the street, perhaps into the past.

"I PLANTED THAT TREE WHEN IT WAS THIS BIG," making an "o" with her index finger and thumb. "I'M VERY PROUD OF MY TREE."

With that, she settled in for a nap in her chair.

KEEPING THINGS SANE, WITH A LITTLE INSANITY

I walk on eggshells all day here. It is a small blessing that Granny is deaf, otherwise she would hear them crunching under my feet as I sneak about the house. I've learned the hard way what reactions brew within her mind when even the slightest change takes place in her home.

You can never forecast an interpretation or response to the lawn being mowed, to a therapist adjusting the wheelchair, to the hydro meter man, or something as simple as a vehicle turning around in our laneway. Things are unpredictable and often quite disturbing for the both of us. Her mind is a funny thing, it will circle the same thought over and over until it almost short-circuits and manifests itself in physical behaviours that are all but pleasant, once again, for both of us.

So, I sneak the furnace man in during bath time. It must seem ridiculous for those who are doing the sneaking, but generally people are sympathetic and understanding of this nasty disease. Those who aren't can go to hell. Being sneaky saves me hours of hair-raising angst, not to mention the frustration of re-explaining the same thought for hours, even days.

I suffered for months with a whacked-out washing machine, due to the logistics of having the old one removed and the new one delivered without her seeing. We managed to keep Granny occupied in her bedroom for the time it took to whisk the machines in and out of the house. What she doesn't know won't hurt her. That is the premise I work on. What she does know, she may not understand, which may cause a kafuffle as her gears try to grasp, or refuse to grasp, the change.

The few times she saw me bring in the groceries were enough to let me know that it upset her. She doesn't want me buying anything and insisted on paying for them, once again, over and over, all the day through, until her purse was empty. I stash the funds in the cupboard and give her the money when she realizes that she's broke. She's pays me again and insists that I'm lying when I tell her that she already paid for the groceries. As thoughtful as she is, it is annoying to spend the day moving money from one place to the other and I no longer let her see the groceries enter the house. I sneak them in, over the eggshells and through the back door.

So I really don't know what I was thinking when I tried to bring my bed frame into the house. I was thinking selfishly of myself; after sleeping for months on my mattress on the floor, I thought that a bed would be fabulous. I had planned to bring it in when she was sleeping, but it wouldn't fit through the door. Logistics, logistics. I had twenty-five minutes to take the bed apart and get it in while the bath lady was there to occupy and distract Granny. Fariel decided to help carry the pieces to my room.

I knew we should have used the grocery door, but things happened too quickly. Granny freaked when the headboard entered the living room. There was no way that any strange piece of furniture was going into her home. You could see she was going to blow a fuse. I've learned to just leave her alone in these times of angst; however, she tried to get up by herself, a precarious attempt to teeter into the wheelchair while taking the brakes off from a standing position.

I went to assist her, to keep her from falling. She wanted no help and made it clear as she wound up and slapped me straight in the face, hard enough to draw tears to my eyes. Her arms were flapping blindly as she wobbled on unsteady feet. Fariel arrived to help me and received a whack of her own. I gave her a little slap on the arm, not to hurt her but to bring her back to reality. She was totally out of control and very upset with me. I was pretty upset myself. Fariel did her best to calm her down before she left. Pissed off, she kicked me out of the house. She is the queen bee here and generally gets her way. I was afraid to go into the living room, so I left a note on her wheelchair apologizing, but also explaining the situation and my feelings.

After a snooze, she awoke pleasant and hungry. We had a light lunch and did the dishes together. I explained that I was leaving for the weekend, in an hour or so. She knew what had happened but didn't know how to verbalize her feelings. They came out as tears. We cried together and hugged and kissed. She begged me to stay, but I was emotionally drained and knew I wouldn't have the right energy to keep her engaged in the way she needs.

I needed to disappear and lick my wounds.

I understood her frustration. I could see that these outbursts are her only means of expressing dissatisfaction, confusion, and her lack of control in her world. I'm not ignorant—but I am human, and my feelings were hurt, even if in my mind I knew that I needn't be.

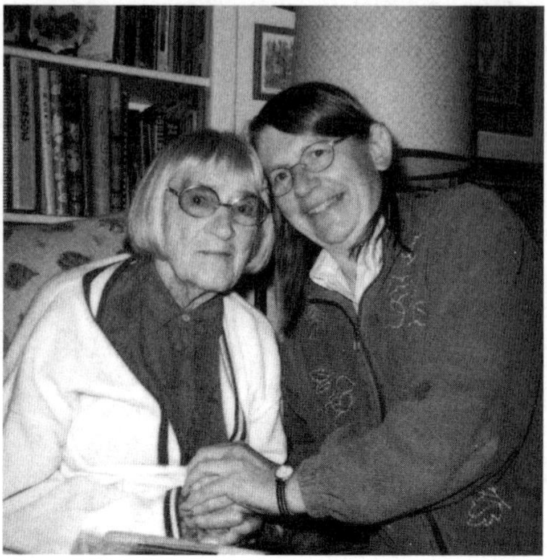

Lenore and Dr. Louise Coulombe

Beyond the day-to-day frustrations of bending in the winds of Alzheimer's, I am exhausted with the system and trying to find help in places where no help is available.

Our biggest blessing is our doctor, Louise Coulombe, who is grounded and straightforward. I have no patience to beat around any bushes and neither does she.

In the fine print, I am scared.

I am so scared, sometimes, at what the future holds for us. I fight sometimes to remain positive and to take everything with yet another grain of salt. I know that these outbursts are only outbursts and not reflecting Granny as she truly is. I also know that she saves them for me—we always hurt those who are closest to us. Nonetheless, I am worried.

I am hoping for a strong rock to stand on.

And a good wind to blow away these worries.

A wind that blows at my back.

And a few answers would be nice.

Answers without questions, please.

The fluid of the moment is sometimes a flood.

I am a chameleon of coping; watch me change my spots.

PLANNING THE LONG-AWAITED GETAWAY

Six days of swimming, eating, sleeping, yoga, and guitar playing has proved to be rejuvenating. It was my longest break in six months, half a year of working—"on call"—500 hours a month. Yes, this seems entirely excessive (the work hours, not the time off). The escape time had made me realize just how freakin' tired I was, am, and will be if I keep this pace up any longer. Naturally, I am a wee bit nervous returning home. My last day with Granny involved hitting, and I wonder if she will be tolerable or aggressive.

Granny is super glad to see me; whew! Our first day was a gallivant of cheer. Fariel arrived at 8:56 a.m. with her smile and while Granny was in the bath, I sneaked my luggage into the house. Someone has swept up some of the eggshells, I'm happy to see. It must have been Laura—she knows how tired I have been getting from stepping over them.

It will be a hectic few days for me. I have been planning a BIG GETAWAY, an intricately scheduled escape, a manifestation of a need to get the hell out of here and do some things for myself, like make some money and hike to the top of as many hills as I can to yodel and hoot my freedom warrior cry. I've scheduled four different ladies, plus the bath ladies; there will be many different faces, unfortunately, as Fariel will also be vacationing. I have organized an unprecedented 700 hours of care for Granny.

Yes, it will be expensive. There are a few alternatives. The first being subsidized respite in an institutional setting, where you pack a confused Granny up and drop her off at a "home." Just leave her a note that says you'll be back in two weeks—fourteen days—and hope to God she doesn't pick up the flu or fall and break something in the confusion of *where the heck am I? Where did Heather go? Am I going to die here?* What will she have forgotten by the time I pick her up?

Who will drop her off? How heavy-hearted will she be? How scared? How confused? How many tears will I shed on my way to the beach? Will the guilt of leaving her in a strange place weigh on my respite? These are questions I don't think I'll ever know the answers to, mostly because of the horrid conclusions to her first stay in Respite Care.

That is option one. It is the only subsidized, government-organized choice we are offered. It's not necessarily a choice, because there are no other subsidized options. Which brings me to the alternative to option one. Don't go away. Stay home and continue to burn out.

Okay, option two might work if I were a martyr, a saint, or just plain crazy. However, I needed to come up with an option three to save my sanity. Option three involves a foundation. I think that's what they are: an organization geared for people like me and people like Granny. Alzheimer's patients and their caregivers can hoot even louder when they meet one of the wonderful Baluchon ladies. These women are specifically trained to deal with dementia and give themselves with their whole hearts to their job, their calling. So they come to the patient's home and stay for one week, replacing the caregiver, relieving the caregiver, and being the caregiver. I really can't believe it! They are angels in our darkness, a light at the end of a long, dark tunnel.

We first met Hélène in early April when she bused from Montreal with a graham cracker-crusted flan pie. The glazed berries glistened atop this Granny delight. As it happened, Hélène won her over with personality alone; the pie was a yummy extra. Although our first attempt for me to get away was cancelled due to the April stroke, Hélène was to return in June and again in late July for a week of Respite.

To begin the week, the caregiver spends twenty-four hours with the Baluchoneuse (French for those people who carry their belongings around in a handkerchief on a stick), and then the primary caregiver goes away. She probably is running. Flying. Skipping. Laughing her way wherever she goes that week, this weight of responsibility lifted, making her light as feathers; the relieved caregiver must be wary of blowing away in even the lightest of breezes. The only thing she has to worry about is doing all the things she has wanted to for six months, which can be overwhelming—there are only so many hours in a week.

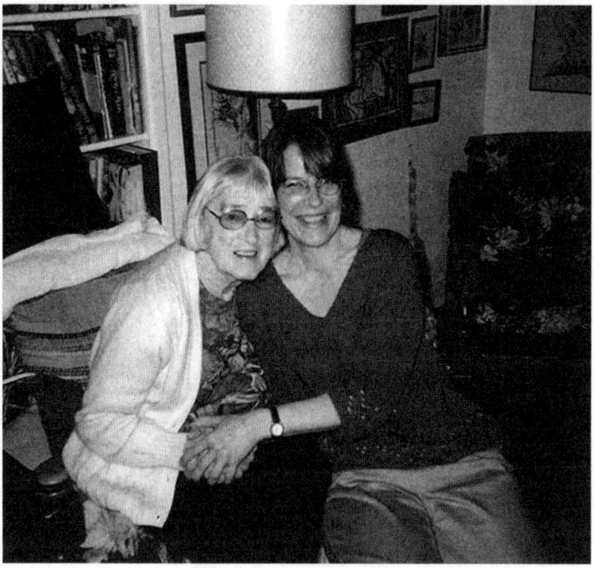

Lenore and Hélène

Needless to say, Hélène is wonderful, and my times away were without worry. If you're ever thinking about giving money away, I suggest that the Baluchon Alzheimer is a fabulous place to donate your bucks. They are not government funded, yet they provide subsidized respite with consciousness to people like us who really need the help. Choosing to care for your loved one at home is a sacrifice and a gift, but without support from people like the Baluchoneuses, it would be an impossibility or a death sentence of sorts.

Once again, we have another solution, another option. Hélène will be part of the 700-hour marathon, a race I had been running alone for months and months, never winning and nothing to lose but my mind.

HÉLÈNE'S TIME WITH GRANNY

Part of the intrigue of the Baluchoneuses is the fact that they take the time to compose a diary of their time with their clients. As the caregiver, it is fabulous to receive these entries to have a bird's eye view of the happenings in your absence. Hélène's journal successfully demonstrates our average day on Iris Street, something I have failed to document in such a way. She has agreed to share her journal and her week with Lenore. The next few pages are a description of her third visit to our home—my second week of respite.

JOURNAL FOR MRS. LENORE SANDERSON
July 27 to August 2, 2005
By Hélène LeBlanc

Reminder: Mrs. Sanderson is deaf but can still talk. We communicate with her by written notes. She has had numerous strokes, therefore her mobility is reduced. She can still walk short distances and manage a few stairs. She uses a wheelchair. I had stayed one week with Mrs. Sanderson from June 5th to the 12th, 2005.

I find her weaker and more sleepy this time. She is more incontinent, not asking for the bathroom, but doing it in the toilet from time to time. Her speech is laborious. She has a hard time sleeping at night because of constant ringing in her ears.

Her granddaughter, Heather, is her main caregiver. She is away working for a few weeks. Laura, Betty, and myself will be staying with Mrs. Sanderson during her absence.

Wednesday, July 27, 2005

I arrive at the Sanderson's around 11 a.m. I am welcomed by Lenore, Fariel (the bath lady), and Laura, who has stayed with Lenore the past few days. Laura is a university student who is also a friend of the family. She had been working as a caregiver for the family this summer. She brings me up to date on Lenore's care. The main change is the re-occurrence of the ringing in the ears. It has happened the last couple of days and had distressed Lenore every time. She tells me to avoid giving Lenore beans, which make her feel uncomfortable.

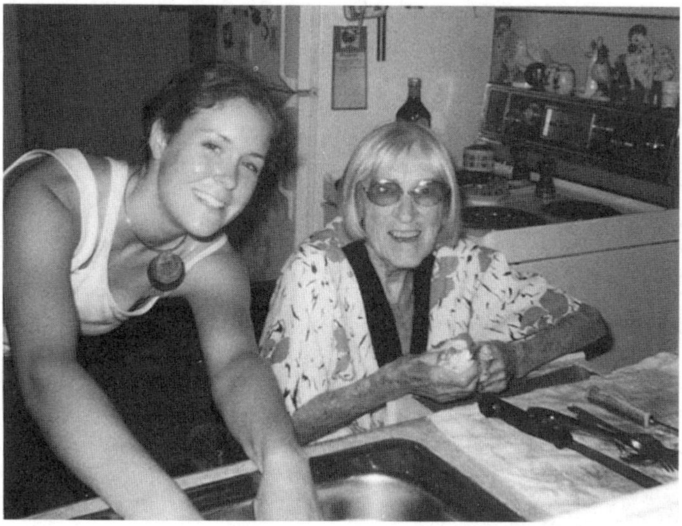

Laura and Lenore

Lenore welcomes me with a smile and is pleased to see me. I'm not sure if she recognizes me but the feelings that we shared are still present.

We have a light lunch and a car ride afterwards. She treats me to ice cream. We have a good time. A good supper, thoroughly enjoyed by both of us. We do the dishes together as always.

Around 7 p.m., she says to me that her ears are ringing. She suggests a car ride but that does not help. She seems very uncomfortable. I give her two Tylenol 3™, we do the bed routine.

She sleeps soundly until 4:30 a.m. and then the ringing starts again. I give her one Tylenol Extra Strength™ and four drops of Rescue Remedy (a homeopathic liquid). At 5:00 a.m. she needs a change and I give her four drops of Rescue Remedy because her ears are still ringing. She sleeps until the bath lady comes in.

Thursday, July 28, 2005

She has a good relaxing morning after the bath and breakfast. I go shopping while Fariel takes care of her. I make sure that I come in with the groceries through a different door. She wants to pay for everything and gets upset when things are brought to the house and she feels she has not paid for them.

I talk to Dr. Coulombe this morning to find out a bit more about the ringing ears. It is part of her disease, she tells me, especially the multiple strokes. It comes and goes and there is not much to do to prevent it. The course of action is as stated in Heather's notes: one Tylenol Extra Strength™ or one Advil™ when symptoms appear. I ask her about the other medications like Tylenol 3™ and sleeping pills; she tells me not to give it to her—just the Ataven™ if she becomes aggressive.

She is upset that she was asleep when Fariel left. She does not remember who the lady is (her regular bath lady), does not remember having a bath and breakfast. I have noticed that her speech is more slurred and that she searches for words at times. I have to watch her because she tries to get out of her chair by herself while I am I in the kitchen. Her short-term memory is affected, since she asks the same questions two or three times. She is nevertheless aware of her limitations and a bit more resigned to the situation.

We have a good lunch and relax on the swing outside in the afternoon. She tells me that she is so happy that her ears are not ringing right now. She tells me that yesterday was awful, ringing and ringing . . . She is relaxed and content. We have a good chat.

At 6 p.m., she is very upset; her ears are ringing as we are preparing supper. I give her one Tylenol Extra Strength™ and invite her to sit in the living room. She does. She also asks me why this is happening now and was not happening when we were outside. I give her a can of Ensure™ (chocolate flavour) and she drinks it well.

Around 7 p.m., she is feeling better. She has a bowl of yogurt and cookies. And is so elated to feel better that she suggests we go on a car ride. We have a beautiful drive on the parkway. There is a beautiful sunset on the river. She is so appreciative of the drive that she gives me some money for gas. I accept it and will put it back in the pot in the cupboard.

We arrive home around 9 p.m. and get ready for bed. Around 12:30 a.m., her ears start ringing, and I give her one Tylenol™. She says that it is louder and louder, driving her crazy, and could I do something. I give her one tablespoon of Children's Gravol™ and four drops of Rescue Remedy. She is in distress and I feel helpless. She somewhat calms down and falls asleep.

At 2:30 a.m., her ears are still ringing, so I give her another Tylenol™ since I can give her one or two every four hours. At 4:30 a.m., she asks to be changed and also says that her ears are still ringing. I give her one tablespoon of Children's Gravol™. She falls asleep shortly afterwards.

Friday, July 29, 2005

She is awake when the bath lady comes in. Even though it's not Fariel, she recognizes that this lady will give her a bath. She is happy and relieved to see me. I can really sense that. I run some errands, do the laundry, and write in my journal while the bath lady is here.

She is bright and alert after her bath. I find her speech more laborious this time. She has more difficulty enunciating. She sometimes has a hard time finding the words and gives up with a smile when she can't find it. She is happy that I am staying. She has a good lunch and is very appreciative.

Around 2 p.m., we set off for Commissioner's Park near Dow's Lake. We have a wonderful stroll and admire all the magnificent flower beds. She is elated. We go for non-alcoholic Margaritas in Dow's Lake Pavilion. Her face has changed a bit. When we get ready to climb in the car she has bumped her elbow, and the mood has certainly changed. We make it home and sitting in her living room chair, she is agitated. I give her one Tylenol Extra Strength™. She is looking for her keys and tells me that I'd better find them when I suggest that I look for them. This is a big change. I don't think I have seen her so cross. She settles down but her ears are ringing and she is upset. I give her a can of Ensure™ (chocolate flavour), and she drinks some of it and it seems to soothe her. She suggests that we have supper; she says that it may help get rid of the ringing ears.

She eats well, and we do the dishes afterwards. She tells me again how she appreciates the long walk we had along the parkway and the beautiful flowers. She regrets having the ringing ears and wonders why it did not occur during the walk. She also worries that there might have been alcohol in our drinks at the restaurant. I reassure her that it is impossible.

We have a long conversation during the evening. She tells me about her travels, the names of the different countries she visited. She talks about her father, her husband, and about a friend who is a painter. I talk to her about my plans for going back to school at McGill University.

Around 9 p.m., we go to bed. No ringing ears but I give her one tablespoon of Children's Gravol™ and she soon falls asleep.

Saturday, July 30, 2005

She sleeps soundly until about 8:15 a.m. when I go to tell her good morning. I had checked her regularly all through the night. She rests in the living room after her bath. I find that she is pale and tired.

We have a good lunch of chicken salad on a bun. We make the sandwiches ourselves at the table, which she seems to like. Dessert: fruit salad and a teaspoon of whipped cream, again a big success. Afterwards, she helps with dishes and the laundry.

She rests some more in the afternoon. She does not feel like going outside. She does not have her usual level of energy and enthusiasm. When she wakes up from a nap, I invite her to the kitchen. She peels the apples that will go in the apple sauce. She eats a snack. Then she tells me that she feels hot. She looks a bit flushed. Returning to the living room, she tells me that she has a headache. I give her one Tylenol™, put a damp cloth on her forehead, and put the air conditioning on.

We have supper around 7 p.m. She eats with appetite and is feeling better. After doing the dishes, we go outside and water the plants. We sit in the swing and chat. She remembers about me going to McGill University. Laura calls us to say "Hi!" and tells me to give a big kiss to Lenore for her. I tell that to Lenore; she is not sure who Laura is. I get the photo album and show her the picture and then she remembers. She also recognizes Laura's dad in one of the pictures but less the other people. She tells me with a sigh: "My memory is not so good anymore." She talks about the vines that are in disarray on the side wall. "Maybe," she tells me, "we should remove them." She regrets not to be able to do the things she used to do like taking care of her house and yard. I tell her how she took good care of her house, which is solid and well-kept. She tells me that she is really proud of her house.

We go to bed around 9 p.m. and I give her one tablespoon of Gravol™ as usual. No ringing ears tonight; she is very calm and content. She rings her bell shortly after being in bed, to tell me that I forgot to put the bedside railing up.

She sleeps well until 2:45 a.m.; she has a headache and her back hurts. I change her and give her one Tylenol™. At 3 a.m., she rings again and tells me she cannot sleep and could I give her something. I give her four drops of Rescue Remedy. I put a facecloth on her forehead and put an extra blanket over her. She often does not remember that she just had some medication. It is difficult to convince her otherwise. She falls asleep afterwards.

Sunday, July 31, 2005

She is sleeping when Fariel comes in. She has her bath and breakfast and rests in the living room. Quiet morning.

She eats well at lunch. Early afternoon, we go for a ride. She is so happy for the ride. We go watch the boats at the marina of Aylmer and have a snack on the island by Champlain's Bridge, admiring the view. We return home after about an hour and a half out. It seems like the right amount of time for an activity. She does not get too tired. She suggests that we go out for supper. I kindly decline. She is not too happy, and I realize why a bit late. She likes to treat people out, because she feels there is nothing in the fridge. She no longer cooks much, therefore she feels she is not being a good hostess.

She does not eat much supper and moves towards the sink to do dishes without wanting dessert. I believe she is still upset with me for refusing her dinner invitation. Returning in the living room, I ask her if she would like to go on a car ride. The answer is a resounding YES. We go for ice cream, her treat, and I think I am forgiven. She is so happy for our second car ride.

We have a good bedtime routine. I give her one tablespoon of Gravol™. She asks me if that will help her sleep. I tell her it will. She rings her bell at 12:15 a.m. and tells me she cannot sleep and could I give her something; one Tylenol™; same thing at 4:15 a.m., plus a change, plus a facecloth on her forehead. She sleeps soundly until morning.

I have a hard time falling back asleep myself after each time and I am wondering how Heather does it if she is awakened two or three times a night and then having to go about her daily routine. When Lenore wakes up in the night, she sounds helpless and supplicant. As mentioned, she asks for medication one minute after she had just had some.

Monday, August 1, 2005

Lenore is still asleep when the bath lady comes in. She has her bath and breakfast and then rests in the living room.

We have a good lunch, do dishes, and then fold laundry. I ask her if she wants to sit outside; she tells me that she does not want to. She is very quiet, observing the action in the birdhouse and on the street. Around 3 p.m., she suggests that we go out for supper. We then set off for a car ride and then stop at Montana's Restaurant for supper. She orders a coffee (not a good idea . . . more on that later). We have a good supper and dessert and . . . no dishes to do. She is very happy.

We return home and sit outside for a while. I rearrange (with her permission) the flower pots so she can have a better view of them. She likes it but despairs that once I am gone she will not be able to water them and they will all die. Despite my reassurances, she is convinced otherwise. She expresses her loss of independence and capacities to take care of her house and her flowers.

I suggest that we go for a car ride, and she enthusiastically agrees. The car ride cheers her up and she thanks me profusely. We return home to sit outside and go to bed around 9:00 p.m.

That is when the afternoon coffee comes to haunt us. At 11 p.m., four drops of Rescue Remedy to sleep, 12:30 a.m., one

Tylenol Extra Strength for ringing ears, at 3:00 a.m., one tablespoon of Gravol™, at 3:30 a.m., four drops of Rescue Remedy for sleep. At one point she even sits up in her bed in an attempt to go to the bathroom by herself; fortunately the bed railing prevents her from doing so. I bring her to the bathroom and change her. I suggest to pull her blanket up: *No!* to put a facecloth on her forehead: *No! That won't help!* Finally, I turn off the nightlight and put on the bathroom light. Her room is dark but there is light in the hallway. She falls asleep around 4 a.m.

Tuesday, August 2, 2005

She wakes up shortly before the bath lady comes in. I go to wish her good morning. She apologizes for keeping me up last night. I give her a big hug and tell her that it was not her fault. She has her bath and then rests in living room.

Kathy, the visiting nurse, arrives at 11:00 a.m. She takes Lenore's blood pressure and asks some questions about how she is doing. Lenore says that her elbow bothers her at times. Lenore is very calm all through the visit. She trusts the medical professionals, they project an aura of authority and she trusts their advice. I sense her to be more fragile and vulnerable, therefore needing reassurance from the medical profession in curing or at least alleviating the pain when it occurs. After the nurse's visit, she thanks me for answering the nurse's questions. Kathy also suggested to practise walking with Lenore, either using the walker or walking with her to keep her mobile.

We have a good lunch that she helps prepare. It is very hot and humid today. We have the air conditioning on, so we chat in the living room for a while. We have a little snack in mid-afternoon. I tell her about Barb's visit and that she will be with her this evening. She is sad and a bit distraught that I am leaving. *So soon, changes, changes . . .* She remembers that I am going back to school and back to Montreal; nevertheless it is hard to say goodbye.
I tell her that she is a very special lady and that I will have her in my heart. "I will miss you," she says. "I will miss you, too."

I am back in Montreal as I am writing these lines. I realize that it may be the last time that I would see Lenore. When you meet someone that has attained the venerable age of 93 years old, the first encounter may be the last. I did not want to think about it during my stay but the thought crossed my mind from time to time. Right now, it brings a lump to my throat and a clunk in my heart. I know also that for Lenore it is a difficult thing having to say goodbye to the ones she meets, as she really puts her heart in meeting and pleasing people during their stay with her.

SLEEP

As you can see by Hélène's journal, we couldn't rest easy in the echoes of Granny's ringing head. I am certain that the hardest part of this whole commitment is the lack of sleep and the inability to alleviate her suffering.

When I first moved here, sleep was just something to tease yourself with. Granny was still able to get out of bed by herself—not safely, mind you—and she would get up a multitude of times every night to pee and do obscure things about the house, like check the locks or take the cake out of the oven. After the big April stroke, not much would stir her slumber. This change was actually disturbing—at times more disturbing than not having any sleep—and I'd sometimes think she was dead with her very irregular breathing.

The hospital bed is a blessing. If you've got a patient who wanders, invest your cash into a bed with rails; it might save you an adventure to the hospital late at night, or at least a small part of your sanity. Be prepared, however, for an adjustment period—people don't like to be trapped in their own bed—but after a month of aggressive midnight rail shaking, they are bound to accept these hindrances; they may even ring their bell to remind you that you forgot to put the bars up. It makes Granny feel good when other people forget and she has to remind them. Lucky for me, any of my absentmindedness is a pat on the back for Granny.

Since the June coma-stroke, Granny is ringing—her head and her bell—several times every night, usually just as you are drifting off. She is also urinating quite a lot more, which I find strange, so now I have been changing her before I go to bed. She has been tuckered out by 7:30 in the evening, making it difficult to change her into her pyjamas. She gets a wee bit emotional every night; she still wants to "not wake up!" But I think she is terrified, and I think that lying down makes her head ache with pressure. I set my alarm for the middle of the night, just in case she has a restful night. I don't want to miss changing her to keep her skin from breaking down.

The last thing in the world we want—well, one of the last things—is a diaper rash. I get up extra early in the morning, before sunrise, to do it again. If the daylight has beaten me out of bed, then when I go to change her, she thinks it's time to get up. "YOU JUST ARRIVED FROM WILNO? LET'S GO FOR LUNCH!" is a terribly frustrating way to start the day. Two hours of, "WHERE'S THE BATH LADY? SHE'S LATE!" can also make your mind turn into goo, even if you got an unprecedented five-hour slumber in. So, I sneak in under the cover of darkness, curtains drawn, lights low, and hope she doesn't realize that it's me who is washing her.

Sometimes, having her granddaughter helping her in such a private way brings her to tears. Sobbing, she will wail endlessly until she falls asleep or gives herself a pride headache. As much as she needs comfort at this time, I've discovered that nine times out of ten, it is best to let her work it out by herself—in this case, my sympathy can only make matters worse.

Hélène wondered how I manage, with all these sleepless nights, and quite honestly, I cannot tell you how. Perhaps I am young enough to take it. Some days I can barely manage to drag myself around the house, let alone Granny, and coincidentally, those are usually her bad days, where she is demanding and impatient—and tipsy. I try to stretch as much as possible, because on tired days, we're both tired, and the fall risk factor is high. I have to be prepared, always, to catch her or I risk hurting myself. I have a bit of a sore hip from hoisting her, and a sore shoulder, too, from compensating for my hip. I do have well-toned arms and legs, though. People ask me if I work out at a gym and I tell them, no, I do Ashtanga Yoga and lift an old lady and push her around the neighbourhood in a wheelchair—a well-rounded workout, to say the least.

My only answer to the "how do you manage" question is: I just do. I anticipate every second weekend, when Betty comes and I retreat to her quiet house to sleep and rest.

Without Betty, my safety net, I would already have collapsed into my own hospital bed, having succumbed to exhaustion; fatigued and listless. So that, my friend, is how I manage, I keep my sights on the end of the tunnel, where the light is—not so far in the future that it appears blurry—and in times of sleep deprivation I think to myself: I will sleep next weekend, I will sleep next weekend, I will sleep, I will.

NOW AND ZEN

For Christmas, Granny received the only one-day calendar that had big numbers and days on it. The standard calendar was starting to confuse her, but she still desired to keep track of the day of the week, and the year. The year is an important part of the date if you're floating through an altered time dimension.

It is a Zen calendar, filled mostly with proverbs, isolated and obscure thoughts, enlightenments, and poetry that are generally far out of the mental grasp of Granny. The calendar was a good suggestion but too confusing for her to understand and utilize as a reminder of a new day, even one day at a time.

So the story goes: I opened it up for New Year's 2005, before my first night out on the town since I moved in with Granny in my crash course in caregiving. January 1. And this is what it said:

"All who enter here should be concerned with the matters of life and death."

A little thought to bring with me out dancing, a heavy thought on the night of resolutions. A good thought to drown with a fancy drink and some funky music. It was a deep and almost dreary thought, not one to display to ninety-two-year-old eyes. Fair warning? Time will tell, as it always does.

TWO RIDES!

Today we had two drives, "TWO RIDES!"—something that both pleased and excited Granny beyond belief. We have a favourite drive—it's my favourite, anyway, and Granny grooves on it, too. It isn't a long drive, saving on gas, but it can turn into a long outing with a bag of stale bread and eyes for a sunset. We hit the parkway, and drive along the river to the bridge to Quebec. This is a double bonus, as Granny is thrilled to visit another province any day of the week. If it's cool enough, warm enough, and dry enough, we can take the wheelchair for a cruise and stroll along the shores of the Ottawa River. Driving, however, is Granny's favourite pastime. We stop in the park on the bridge and assist in further taming the wild life as we tempt them to our car with honey mustard sesame sticks and the like. I can't remember where we went on the second drive but it really doesn't matter. Maybe we went to the lookout at the Experimental Gardens, overlooking the arboretum.

The *where* is redundant but the thank-yous are abundant. She thanked me repetitively all night. "TWO RIDES IN ONE DAY!" was the last thing she said to me that night; she even mumbled that phrase in her sleep. Simply simple: easy to please, I like that, too.

REGRETFULLY WITHDRAWING

When we say, "they say," we usually are referring to an unwritten truth or rule. When I say, "they say," in this instance, I am referring to an unwritten rule, not a truth, and not particularly even a rule but a circumstance of living in this day and age.

They say you can't beat the system. When I first appealed for more funding for Granny's care—for my freedom and peace of mind so that I don't wind up crying my eyes out on dance floors everywhere—I had a hint of hope. I hoped for some compassion for the road we are on, a beautiful road, a bumpy road, a rocky trail, to say the least. Nevertheless, I was a wee bit foolish to think it would be an easy breeze to sway the system. I first spent months looking for help, then I spent weeks looking for help to look for help, only to have my eyes pried open by the stark reality: the system has no loopholes set up for people in our situation. We are in another reality altogether. The loopholes that the system has are designed so that people appealing for help eventually give up or sink 150,000 dollars into a Supreme Court proceeding. I'll tell you, with that kind of cash on hand, I wouldn't *need* outside help.

I'm a pretty thorough individual. I read the Long-Term Care Act, The Practice and Procedures Act, the Red Tape Reduction Act, and a multitude of other legal documents—hundreds of pages—to ascertain that even if Granny isn't capable of living alone, she is capable of deciding what she wants. I learned that our community care provider, the organization we were appealing to, had no jurisdiction to provide us with any more help than the fifteen hours a week we already had. In order to appeal to the next level, we had to lose at this level and appeal the appeal. According to the Long Term Care Act, there is a provision where the Minister of Health can grant funding to individuals, as he or she sees fit. I am told that this would be my only avenue for assistance, apart from a Supreme Court case, which would undoubtedly take longer than Granny had left on this earth and require more energy than I had.

To make a long story short, there were several pre-conference telephone hearings, the first being with me, my friend, Lauren, the care service provider, and the mediator from the appeal board. The second was with me, at the hospital, with Granny in a coma, on line with counsel for the MofHLTC (Ministry of Health and Long-Term Care) and the community care service provider, their staff, and the mediator. The final telephone conference included all of the above, plus my counsel, who, on my behalf, withdrew my appeal.

Others before me have fought the system and lost. One gentleman, in particular, won his case. Many organizations backed him up with funding for counsel, rights groups everywhere rallied behind him, and he won. Although he won, nothing changed; a loophole is a loop. He will probably fight until he is in the grave, costing him his time, his life, the energy and money of advocacy groups, and the time and money of the government—the taxpayers' money, to be more specific—all because these Acts and Regulations have been designed to send us spinning in circles.

Anyway, it has been a relief in the end not to think about it. I have, to date, written two letters to the current Minister of Health, both invitations: one to high tea with me and Granny and the other to talk with me about care solutions that will benefit society as a whole. There was a third letter, but it came back due to insufficient postage; I thought letters to Queen's Park were free to mail, but it seems only if they are under a certain weight. I never mailed that one and have yet to hear back with any RSVPs for tea and cookies on Iris Street.

PIGGIE SITTING

My niece, Brittany, has become a regular part of our lives—a special treat for both Granny and myself. Once a week, we pick her up after school. With guitar in hand, she brings with her an appetite for ice cream and about three tons of joy to our home.

"ARE WE GOING TO GET THE LITTLE ONE? . . . WE'RE GETTING THE WEE ONE!" is what you would hear if you were in our car for the twenty minutes it takes to get to the east end of the city.

Brittany writes notes while I drive, and while I make supper. Granny can hardly take her eyes off her "wee beauty" as she fascinates us with crafts, charm, and hip-hop dancing.

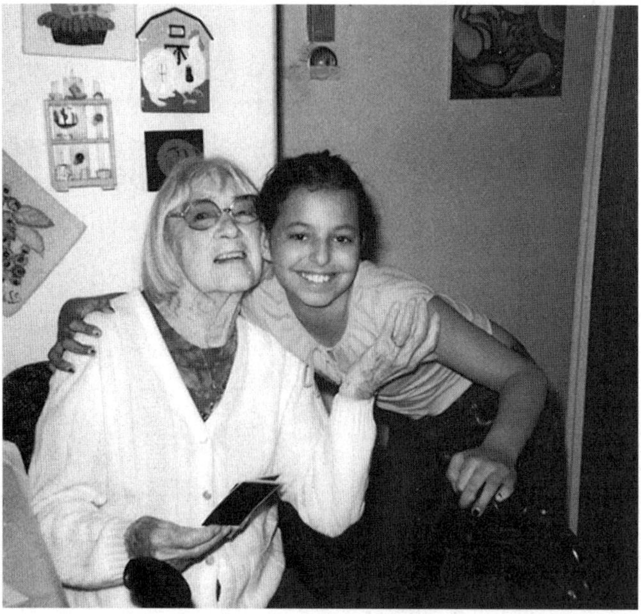

Lenore with great-granddaughter Brittany

Brittany has a guinea pig. His name is Bernie, and as far as rodents go, he is pretty cute and affectionate. We were pig-sitting for two weeks during summer vacation. I thought it would be a fun distraction for us; the heat had been oppressive and we were housebound and needing internal stimulation. Sometimes Bernie was the cat's meow, but often he was the plague, turning our home "INTO WILD KINGDOM!"

On the sunny side, he was hours of fun, causing copious amounts of giggling as Granny hand fed him radicchio and arugula. It turns out that Granny had always wanted a guinea pig. Not just any guinea pig, either. She wanted a specific guinea pig that was at the Carlingwood mall. In those days, she would go every day to Sears, presumably to score with shoe sales. With her step counter on, she'd wander thousands of steps around the mall and stop for a coffee break right in front of the pet store. That is where she saw the piggie of her dreams. My mom recalls: "She wanted THAT guinea pig. She talked about him for months. She'd visit it every day. One day the guinea pig was gone—she never spoke of it again. And never wanted another one!"

That was obviously a very special pig, because Bernie didn't cut it. Some days, she'd make her horrid face and flap her hands in front of her when I took him out for a feeding. For better or worse, Bernie was worth his weight in celery for the hours that he kept Granny happy in her hands. The other day I asked her if she missed Bernie the guinea pig. She looked around, just to make sure no one was in hearing range, looked at me and made a face, a face of disgust and displeasure. "Not a bit," she confessed when she was certain that no offence would be taken.

I think that she was even being gracious with a rodent. Really, what a woman! Her sense of dignity will see her through the often graceless moments of this disease. A little grace can go a long way; it can see us through.

REFLECTING IN WATER

I can't believe what this break is doing to my head. I haven't had the time or the will to process the past months. I really don't know how I've been managing. I haven't even become a coffee junkie or an alcoholic, small wonder.

But WOW, it is insane to think about not thinking and only doing for me. Me, first, like a selfish child instead of a selfless adult. Not thinking is meditating, in one form or other. It is fundamentally important to have uninterrupted nothing; to have this nothing floating internally. How do we stop the hammering around our skulls, the creeping thoughts or wandering ponderances that venture in and linger? I knew that I had to get back to just looking out my eyes, not preparing or recovering, just being; calm and content. It took a few days to really settle down and begin to become myself again. It's not that I lost myself in so many words, but I lost some little pieces that make everything run smoothly.

It's easy to find this peace, my inner quiet, underwater. Submerged in August waters is an awesome way to forget the world and begin to selfishly think only of myself and stop this hammering of:

What do I want?
How can I facilitate my needs?
How can I have time for myself?
How can I keep this peace at times of extreme adversity?
Whom can I count on to help us?
Where do I find this help?

The questions are many and the time is short. Days fly by, one by one, sunrise, sunset, starshine, moonset.

Reflecting, I have learned so much: both practical knowledge and inner knowing, an understanding that I might have earlier claimed, but not to this extent. They say you acquire knowledge from a book and wisdom from experience. This experience kicked my wise ass into a new light of understanding, a gift I am told will only truly show its face in the years to come, when this phase of my life has become a closed chapter. I guess that that is why it is called reflecting: you have to be on the other side to have a reflection—you can't be immersed, or submersed, for that matter. Perspective is everything, and hindsight is twenty-twenty. I can foresee that hindsight, but I can't see how it will perceive this fragment of my life.

Thankfully, I've learned to trust the care of the ladies that stay with Granny. I believe that everything will always work out for the best, even if the road is long and hard, even if it's uphill and we're tired, or steeply downhill and we can't slow down. It has taken eight months to devise this system I have—running smoothly, I must add, just to pat myself on the back.

It's important to pat yourself on the back.

Only a few minor disturbances have occurred in my absence. The biggest one involved the air conditioner repairman, so it was an expected and necessary evil. Oh, I nearly forgot, because it wasn't my problem, I'll bet. One of the temporary bath ladies left before her shift was over—before Laura got home! Laura said that a shoeless Lenore was rolling herself around the house, muttering, "I'm so confused. I'm so confused."

Laura is assertive and articulate. She told me flat-out, "I filed an official complaint. I documented everything on my computer." Laura is smart enough and wise, sweet but strong enough, that she might just be able to change the world when she graduates from university with her political science degree. I'm selfishly glad that I missed this incident. I probably would have said something I would regret later.

The worst thing that Granny and the ladies are facing is the ringing of the ears.

Granny's ears ring and ring. It is so loud that, "IT MIGHT WAKE THE NEIGHBOURS! CAN'T YOU HEAR IT, HEATHER?" she queries.

"No," I admit, shaking my head.

"I CAN'T BELIEVE IT! IT'S SO LOUD! IT'S DRIVING ME CRAZY!" she screams, and holds her head. Sometimes she even sobs. There really is nothing that can be done to quiet the sirens in her mind. It is positively horrible for her and for whoever is trying to keep her content and comfortable. Some nights, sleep will never come to our house, or if it does arrive, it is only enough to tease an exhausted caregiver before she gets up to write a note: "Just be patient, your medicine will start to work soon," which until recently was a lie. Now we have Atavan™ sedatives and they can successfully knock her out cold; a little peace in the storm.

"WOULD YOU JUST MAKE IT STOP!" is a demand more than a request. She can get quite agitated and needs to blame someone for her suffering. I can only imagine the discomfort of a raging, screaming ringing in her head. I can sympathize, but my hands are tied when it comes to a cure. Diagnosis: tinnitus. It's when the olfactory nerve generates its own sound even in the ears of the profoundly deaf, triggered by high blood pressure, infection, antibiotics, caffeine, stress, and drugs—to name a few examples listed in my medical book, which also suggests that we try to find distractions and learn to live with it. Blah, blah, blah, blah.

BLAH.

Ha.

Ha.

Ha.

A SPACE FOR ME

I have finally found a place in the backyard to sit, a place where no one can see me apart from the mourning doves that coo with every breaking day. They are the doves that come to our feeder in Granny's maple. It is a place where the baby monitor works, nestled between two houses, behind a lilac, the cypress and spruce trees blocking windows to the northeast and my mind blocking out the traffic that whirls by, maybe thirty feet behind my back. I am relieved to have found this place. It is as though the trees have grown just to protect me from the world and the eyes that might be watching.

I am a country girl, used to the vast open spaces of the mind and the comfort of nature that embraces me there. I have adjusted to the city, the suburbs, where most of my time is spent, but I often yearn for the sanctity of forest. I have learned to find repose internally—yet another lesson, a gift I have chosen to accept, nurture, and refine.

These are such minute details of life. Funny, how "minute" and *minute* are the same word, with different sounds. A minute is only a minute moment, these fractions adding up to the whole. Time passes so quickly, yet it is these minute minutes that mark the time with crossroads, tribulations, trophies, and tenderness. We are all minutes. We are all minute in grandiose being. All we touch, touches. All we sense, senses. To get all philosophical—we are part of the air. All in all, all is good—even the bad or the difficult, especially if you've found your wee spot, a safe zone where no one can find you, yet you're still here in awareness, free from action and distraction. Here I sit. Here I be.

LOOKING BACK

I remember, indeed I do, many times spent with Granny, throughout my lifetime, going back as far as to when she owned a turquoise station wagon, to a time when I was small enough to curl onto her lap for stories on the big gold carpet, the one she and Donna made.

She would take us, my sister and me, gallivanting through the city, us country bumpkins riding in style with our hip Granny in her bright blue wagon. She would amaze us with museums, malls, and dining out. We'd devise a craft project and zip off to White Rose, stopping for ice cream on the way home before we'd spend the evening creating. Little did I know then, that is what Granny did: zip around and buy stuff, stopping here and there for coffee, treats, and sales. She loved to shop, and more important, she loved to take people shopping. She loved to buy things, and once again, she loved to buy people things.

The queen of sales, she loved a good deal. Especially, she loved to buy sale items from Sears, the only department store she ever had a credit card for. Of a different era, she probably never used the card, but had it just in case she didn't have enough cash in her wallet for those stylish new heels or that fancy sweater.

She would also come to visit us at the farm, where she would follow me around the acreage, snapping photos of my minnow traps and favourite rocks. She'd always say she was a city girl, but boy, did she love nature and all the creatures under the sun. There was no worry about her keeping up, either, because she walked five miles a day until she was eighty; perhaps that is why she's still here, with strong lungs and heart—incredibly fit for ninety-three.

Although I never met my grandfather, she told me plenty of stories about him, in particular about playing tennis and flying with him. He took her out every weekend, even after they separated, for romantic sunset flights.

Not much—well, nothing—could hold my Granny back, not with good friends to travel the world with and inspiration to create and try new things.

Much of what she taught me was by example—by the way she lived her life with spontaneity, independence, and drive. She showed me how working hard, balanced with leisure, friends, and creative outlets, made a person whole and satisfied. *Inspired* is the word; *free spirit*. She showed me how to believe in myself and in the world of opportunities. I learned a great deal about sharing, through her sharing with me. I'm not talking about objects shared or loaned, either, but time and energy. She gave freely of herself, and even as a small child I could see the admiration in the eyes of her friends and acquaintances that I would meet. *Generous* is yet another word.

Some of our moments are captured in snapshots, even Polaroids™ from the camera we are now using to document visitors. For many of these photos, I have no memory of the actual moment—I suppose that the early years of life are quite similar to the latter—we recall the photo but not the when or where. I can certainly comprehend the comfort that Granny's massive collection of albums provide her, and, as of late, the angst she experiences when staring into the pages for forgotten memories, those faces and names erased from her mind. The once often-told stories that accompany the photos are lost, but she still knows that she should know. It must be entirely frustrating for her to be trapped from this history—*herstory*, to be exact. I wish I could remember for her, but of course that would be embarrassing for her; in many ways I think she is willing to let it all go, sit back, and watch the birds at the feeder.

POETRY OF A SONG

Please do what you want with my house.
I can't hear anything, anyhow.
My world's not closing in, but opening up.
Please come in for cookies and a cup.

If I could, I would take pictures of my memories.
But all we've got's the moment—let's go for coffee.
I haven't lost my marbles, they're all just misplaced.
Just yesterday, I couldn't place my best friend's face.
I can't find the word, can't put my finger on it.
But thank you for bringing me home.
You're so beautiful and I'm so tired.

Just do what you want—what makes you happy.
Do what you want with my house.
You know I want to be gone by sunrise.
I just want to die at home where the heart is.
Thank you for bringing me home
Thank you
Thank you
Thank you

FLASH IN THE PAN

One day, Granny asked me, "HOW LONG WILL YOU BE STAYING, HEATHER?"

It may seem like I write my own name for effect, when I quote Granny, but she does say my name often, especially with questions. I think she is reminding herself that she still knows who I am. Which, as you can imagine, is very important to her; to remember, that is, the name of the person she sees every day, the person who happens to be her granddaughter. She does ask the same question, this same question, often, as well, for assurance that I will not leave her.

"HOW LONG WILL YOU BE STAYING, HEATHER?"

Here we go again.

"*I live here.*"

"OH!" pause to ponder.

"HOW LONG WILL YOU BE STAYING?"

"*I live here.*" I point to the last note—they are handy that way.

Another pause in time.

"HOW LONG HAVE YOU LIVED HERE?"

"*Six months.*"

"HOW LONG?"

"*Six months.*"

"SIX MONTHS! WOW!" she exclaimed, shocked.

"I CAN'T BELIEVE IT! SIX MONTHS!"

She said that all day. It was a long six months for her, yet they disappeared as only a flash in the pan. Who could keep track of the time with all that happened? I can scarcely track the time and my mind is fresh and young. Home from the Home with a bladder infection, a bone infection, seizures and strokes, in the hospital twice, deemed palliative, brought home to die, miraculously recovering, taking massive doses of drugs and antibiotics and living in between. It's no wonder that timelines are irrelevant at this point. It certainly blew her mind to find out that I'd been in her home for six months. It was the last thing she said before I kissed her goodnight and the first thing she forgot in the morning.

Perhaps she asked me again the next day just to make sure—an affirmation that she was with good company, someone who would stand by her through thick and thin. Perhaps she doesn't really forget but wants to be reminded—reminded that she is not alone, and that she doesn't have to live with that sinking fear of spending the rest of her life where she knows no one and no one knows her. It is a gift that I am more than willing to give—and I'll give it with gratitude, even if gratitude is something we generally accept. There are no rules here.

HOW DID WE MISS DAVE

Who's Dave, anyway?

Dave is a little magic thrown into West End suburbia. He's a man who has it figured out. By It, I mean life. His time off, to him, is worth more than his time working. How you interpret that is up to you.

He is, nonetheless, a hard worker, who in his spare time salvages metal, stripping copper wires and stashing them in his garage, patiently waiting for copper prices to rise; sort of like playing the stocks. He is a handy man, and was Lenore's handyman for years and years. He is a man of heart, and always remembers Lenore and pops over periodically with gifts, smiles, and pages of pre-written notes. Who the hell takes the time to pre-write notes to a deaf old lady? Obviously, he is a man who cares a lot about Lenore, just a woman down the street. In the past, he would take her for drives to see the Christmas lights and out for coffee. She would even write me letters telling me about Dave's ride. If you have a little old lady on your block, you won't believe the good feeling you can give—and get—by just saying "Hi!" and I hope that reading this will be incentive for you to do just that. Old people are often lonely and really appreciate the kindness of neighbours.

I read that doing a good deed releases endorphins (little happy pain relievers) in our brains; and having a good deed done produces the same euphoric state of mind. What's more, *witnessing* a good deed done has the same effect on our physiology. Keep that in mind, not that we should benefit from helping one another, but we do reap rewards from kindness. Why not? Thanks, Dave. Granny thanks you, too. And she still knows your name and your face. That's a compliment, that's for certain.

VISITORS FROM THE OTHER SIDE

Late-night visitors come to Granny. They are often people that I've never met, often from the other side. Both her parents were in our bubble during her stroke recovery, and last night, her brother Harvey came to her in her dreams. As far as I have understood, Harvey was killed by a train in California, when Lenore was still a young woman, or even a child. In actuality, she has rarely mentioned him to me, another black cloud in her past that I assume she would prefer to forget. She awoke this morning wondering when his birthday is—was, I guess—but no, is: she was in the present with him; he came to her in a dream. She said he went away. "He got tired of waiting," sadness in her voice.

I asked if he went to Heaven, and the face she made said a thousand words. Definitely, he is not in Heaven—he was in her dreams. I have to wonder, sometimes, if these spirits are waiting, perhaps even with impatience, for Lenore to come to their side, and leave this realm of the earthly plain. Contemplating, I wonder if he got fed up waiting some eighty years for his sister to join him. Maybe he's even given up at this point, chosen to be reborn, or whatever spirits choose when they are wherever they are. It all can be very vague, but oh-so real for her, and I wish I could see through her eyes. She seemed so alert this morning—her words clear and her eyes bright. God only knows; indeed, only He would know.

A FRIENDLY VISITOR

If I haven't said it before, then I will say it now, and again later, because these simple truths in life are just that—true, and it is good to remind ourselves of them, if not periodically, then regularly. Little coincidences can really renew my faith that the universe is looking out for us; things always do happen for a reason.

According to her last Geriatric Assessment, in December 2003, Granny was put on a waiting list with the local seniors' community centre for a friendly visitor, a volunteer who is to regularly visit seniors in need of social interaction. I phoned several times over the last months until I finally gave up; there aren't enough volunteers to go around, as the story goes. I'm sure that many a community program is waiting for volunteers. In this busy day and age, we can't really blame people for selfishly keeping their time for themselves or for their own elders who are also in need of visitors.

I made contact with the Friends of Hospice over the summer, and applied for a friendly visitor for Granny, someone to come and give me a break from writing and supervising. As luck would have it, we had a visitor lined up almost immediately. As fate served us, the woman, Marion, turned out to be an old student of Granny's and had fond memories of Lenore, her talents and personality.

They hit it off like a grand slam; granted, at first Granny assumed that I would be leaving and was reserved and suspicious. We ate dinner together, and then I disappeared, periodically appearing to assure her that I was still present, not abandoning her with another stranger—everyone is a stranger when you have Alzheimer's. It is sad, but true. Marion, however, became an instant friend—"SPECIAL KIN," were Granny's words to describe her as I tucked her into bed that night. They spent the evening poring over photo albums, chatting and reminiscing. Marion awoke memories in

Granny that I don't doubt had been sleeping for a long time. Perhaps it was just a lucid day, but my heart tells me that they made a strong connection in those few hours—like magnets attracting—like keys to hidden doors—like the instant magic of pixie dust.

That enchanting powder didn't just affect Granny. I could see in Marion's eyes and by her words and actions that she was as captivated as Granny with this renewed alliance. Granny begged her to come back, please, please.

So now we will have a regular visitor coming, someone who feels fulfilled and fills, sharing time with Granny—and it shows. Granny can sense Marion's joy and thrives on it.

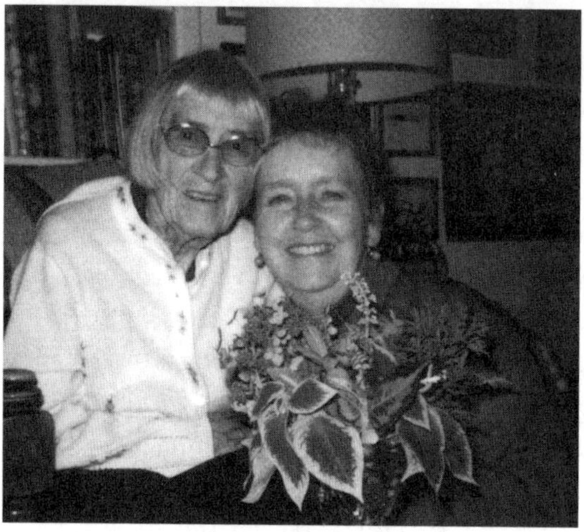

Lenore and Marion

Myself, I sat outside, in my little space, for a good while, free of the baby monitor and the note pad. I even lay in my bed without wondering what was happening in Granny Land. I could hear their laughter drifting down the hall like a far-away radio program. I could tune in or tune out. It's a pleasure to have a choice between being aware or spacing out. The next time Marion comes, next Monday, I will take a long bath and I will luxuriate knowing that the bell won't be ringing beside Granny's bed. I won't be worried that I might miss her call with the water running. I won't emerge dripping into her room with one shaved leg or shampoo still in my hair. Believe it or not, I can hardly wait. It truly is the small things that we can look forward to.

Coincidence or fate—little does it matter on the scale of wonders, especially when an old acquaintance becomes a fresh and welcomed guest in our home and lives.

MORE ABOUT THE TREE

There is one thing that Granny has always felt absolutely terrible about: the leaves from her giant crimson maple that fall each year, marking the seasons in deep maroon wisps of wind. She would have liked to pick up every last one of those leaves, if not for those winds that tend to scatter things like leaves.

If only they would fall straight down to the ground on a still day, then she could scoop them up into bags and keep the neighbourhood neat and tidy. She always felt that the neighbours were disgruntled at the mess that tree left behind. She didn't want any negative feelings to harbour around her, or about her, or to be directed at her tree.

I can scarcely imagine someone cursing that tree, or the old woman who looks out from behind it, but anything is possible, I suppose, in this world of blame.

If, by chance, any of those neighbours are reading this, disgruntled or not, please accept the utmost apologies from Mrs. Iris Street. I assure you, she has spent many sleepless nights over those leaves and the tribulation that proceeds from them as they radiate out into the neighbourhood. She is truly sorry for any inconvenience that they may have caused. She has probably even sprained a wrist or broken an ankle in attempts to stop them from escaping the yard.

On the brighter side, if you let one of those maple keys sprout in your yard, you could cultivate a tree like the one in Mrs. Iris Street's yard. The seeds are viable, and they will grow unless you want to stop them. Perhaps you, too, will peer through the leaves and branches when you grow old, and fear the repercussions of all those damn leaves. Keep in mind that it will probably attract pesky birds and be perfect for hanging Christmas lights in, and perhaps if that tree grows up in your yard, it may very well be a sprout that will become your pride and joy, a comfort and a confirmation that you were here, planted a tree, and left.

GRANNY LOSES HERSELF IN THE PAINTINGS

A small blessing it is, a grand gift it is, to be able to create my art while Granny watches, spellbound by the brushstrokes, mesmerized. I admit, at first I found it difficult to be stared at, like a side-show at the circus, but I've grown accustomed to her eyes on me and really don't mind a bit. It is an activity for both of us, fulfilling two needs in one.

One day I was working on a large painting and it was very difficult for me to see the canvas for my own shadow. It was hard for Granny, too, and she was getting frustrated. Loud sighs cued me to move from her light. "WOULD YOU JUST MOVE YOUR HEAD?" she said, annoyed with me. "YOU'RE IN MY LIGHT!" she complained. *Who's painting the picture*? I giggle to myself.

Finally, with a long sigh, even a moan, she said, "WELL, I MIGHT AS WELL BE WATCHING TELEVISION IF YOU CAN'T KEEP YOUR HEAD OUT OF THE WAY!" She is always straight to the point, isn't she?

Luckily, I switched to acrylic paint in the spring. The oil was frustrating me because of the need to spend constant time at it. It would dry on me, not in the stage I would want, and I'd have to rework the entire piece.

Luckily for Granny, I switched to acrylic paint. We usually have a snack on hand, on the side table between our chairs. My palette, on the day in question, was a takeout container. I had gone to do the laundry and didn't hear from the baby monitor the sound of her reaching and having a snack. When I returned, I can honestly say that I was nearly sick to my stomach when I saw the paint all over Granny's face and hands. She mustn't have much left in the way of taste buds because she was chewing old rubbery paint like a camel, the fresh paint blending into a seriously foul shade of browny-purple. What to do?

“You’re eating paint!” I write.

She was pretty upset when she figured it out—not at eating the paint, but getting it on her hands. I certainly wouldn’t be showing her a mirror. “OOPS,” she casually says and we head to the washroom to brush her teeth and wash the green paint from her nose and chin. She was amazed when she spit out the toothpaste; I’m sure she’d never spit out so much colour.

“You ate paint,” I explained. And that was that. That was the day that I learned to keep my palette out of reach, and that Granny had no sense of taste left. I like it when we learn two things at once; it makes for fewer lessons later. Small blessings are still blessings, and often a good chuckle later in the day, once your stomach stops turning.

Learning to Speak Alzheimer's

This is the title of a must-read book for caregivers, family, and friends dealing with Alzheimer's and dementia. Without these tips, I would have pulled every hair out of my head by now. It's amazing how cueing chores and personal care can allow Granny the pleasure of doing things for herself. I have been putting the paste on her toothbrush and leaving it on the sink, so when she arrives to wash her hands, she knows to begin her ten-minute standard ritual of cleaning, perfectly, her teeth, with toothpaste and not anti-bacterial liquid hand soap.

Little things do matter, like the colour of the wall behind the toilet. These victims face a new way of seeing, where depth perception is lost when contrasts are low. Thankfully I picked up a copy of this book before renovating the bathroom at Iris Street, as it encouraged me to be bold with the wall paint intensity. That is why our washroom is bright salmon orange, perhaps the brightest colour you will ever see on a two a.m. pee break. The experts say that Alzheimer's patients aren't necessarily incontinent, meaning that it's not a physical condition but a mental lapse. They simply forget to go before it's too late—so the theory goes—thus a white throne on a vibrant wall jumps out and reminds, without blatantly saying it in words. Interesting.

The funniest part, for me, about the renovations was that Granny didn't notice the changes at first. It took several days for her to notice the walls and she squealed, "WHAT A LOVELY COLOUR!" but she never noticed that the sink had moved and part of her bedroom closet was missing. She was also oblivious to the fact that her multitude of heeled dress shoes—over a hundred pairs in all—were no longer in the closet, either.

I should correct myself. She was oblivious to this change, but late one night, amidst her dream-talk garbles, these words reached me in my bed clear as day: "WHERE ARE ALL MY SHOES!" she said, as much a question as an exclamation.

I thought for certain that I would be in for it in the morning, back to explaining the safety issues of sauntering about in heels at ninety-two. Come morning, the knowledge of the loss of the shoes was thankfully forgotten, and she didn't protest the Velcro Walkables™ that are now her only sturdy footware.

A bath lady once gave in to Granny's desire to wear flashy shoes. Boy, was Betty upset—it was her day with Granny—when she was helping Granny up and her feet shot out from under her like a cartoon character on a banana peel. Thankfully, no one was hurt. Old ladies fall funny. If you're not always prepared with bent knees, you can risk popping something out of place in your own body, which would certainly cause big troubles in Careville.

Betty said that Granny was almost perturbed at those shoes; why would she be wearing such slippery feet? She has never again asked to change out of those white runners. We do have to polish them periodically to keep her satisfied, which is comical in itself—buffing sneakers, that is.

Instead of wearing fancy shoes to match her fancy clothes, she now prefers casual wear. Some days she will let the bath lady put her in a skirt or dress, but then reality sets in when she sees her feet. She'll sigh and sigh. As the sighs turn to huffs, she will declare, "THESE SHOES DON'T MATCH MY SKIRT!"

And with that, we are off to put on pants.

Mrs. Seto

Today, Granny figured out that I had gone shopping for groceries. I have been dreading this day, but it has arrived with a state of shock for Granny. She is devastated that I would have to buy her groceries—imagine that, your granddaughter coming to visit and filling your fridge. The realization brought her to tears. Not even bubble blowing or birthday sparklers would cheer her from this terrible knowledge. What's even worse is that with the fridge full it leaves no excuse for dining out for every meal during my visit with her.

Changes, changes. A pineapple appearing in the kitchen can cause a whole pile of anxiety for the elderly. So many times, I have used the excuse, "Mrs. Seto brought it over for you!" It is an acceptable explanation for strange fruit and bags of cheese curds. Mrs. Seto had probably brought over these items countless times, in the many years they have been neighbours. Without her consideration and concern, Granny would have certainly found herself in an institution, or the morgue; or more correctly, down at the university having her ears dissected by specialists.

I, too, have relied on Mrs. Seto's kindness and love for my granny, especially when she still lived alone. She would take out the garbage and bring the recycling box back to the house. She'd even slip the science experiments from the refrigerator into the garbage, saving Granny and her guests from food poisoning.

Granny always said, "I raised the neighbourhood!" and this is assuredly true. Mrs. Seto also was a single mother, holding down several jobs to raise her family. I think that her children frequented Lenore's kitchen and company over the years; Nancy, in particular, still visits every Christmas with presents and love. I think that in this day and age we have lost sight of neighbours, perhaps for fear of too much involvement. Mrs. Seto is an exceptional woman, keeping in mind the needs of her friend next door.

She has a key to the front door, and when things started to slip, she would check in with Granny—three times a day! In the morning, she would unlock the door for the bath lady, who would be standing ringing the doorbell, its light fruitlessly flashing in the living room as Granny slumbered on. Between jobs, she would stop in with some food and enjoy a meal in the rooster room. Once Granny had tucked herself in for the night, Mrs. Seto would lock the front door. Granny figured that leaving it unlocked was the only was to ensure that the bath lady would get in the following morning—deductive reasoning.

An unbelievable fact is that this beautiful friendship is maintained without a means of communicating particulars. Mrs. Seto has limited knowledge of reading and writing, so they interact with smiles and gestures, like two foreigners. I must say that they get by wonderfully even without words.

It was Mrs. Seto who responded to the Help-line alarm and discovered Granny on the floor after trying to move the television set with heels on. She confided in me that when the panic button calls came to her, she would proceed next door terrified that she would find Lenore dead in the house somewhere. It is quite a commitment to be the first one called when catastrophe hits, before family and the ambulance, and to conquer the fear of discovering your long-time friend in a broken state or bad way.

Currently, I don't rely on Mrs. Seto's kindness. I feel she has gone beyond the call of duty in the past and I do not want to burden her anymore. But I have a sense of reassurance that our closest neighbour to the kitchen window would be over in a flash if we needed any help—needed anything, for that matter.

Granny always says, "I have such good neighbours!" You have to be a good neighbour to have good neighbours, unless you live in a neighbourhood of saints and angels, which is what good neighbours become to the elderly. Granny forgets now that she was a good neighbour, generous, kind, and thoughtful—she remembers only that she is incapable of helping in ways she would like the wonderful people, the chosen kin, who have assisted her over the years. Some days I wish her sense of dignity weren't so infallible—that she could accept help without guilt—but her dignity is the last thing that I will take away from her; the last thing she will surrender.

BEWARE OF THOSE WHO KNOW TOO MUCH

This is just a quick note to prepare you for the fact that even the smartest individuals, whose job it is to assist in decision making and planning, really don't know anything more than their job. Keep in mind that if you are the caregiver, family member, or best friend, you undoubtedly know more about the person in question than anyone else. Trust your instincts and be assertive.

This is particularly true when it comes to the social workers in the hospitals. In my opinion, which may not reflect anything more than my feelings, the social worker's job is to get people out of the hospital, by whatever means. They are not doctors and should not speak as doctors. In fact, they should just say it like it is, without trying to scare people into placing their loved ones into long-term care.

This is my little insight that I picked up in hindsight, after our social worker told me that Granny would never walk again. "But she broke her *elbow*," I protested. Anyway, she freaked me out, and with no true means of actually determining this crippling fact—they hadn't even tried to get her out of bed! Now it is almost a year later, and even after several strokes, Granny can walk; she can even go up the three stairs that lead through the front door.

So if you're a social worker, keep in mind that your forecasts for the future are merely personal opinions and not the straight goods. Indeed, no one can be prepared for everything, but already upset families need not hear a misdiagnosis from an unqualified voice, even if the aim is to get a fire going under their butts to make these hard-core decisions, and quickly, because the hospital needs the bed and time's a-wastin'.

Don't let anyone push you into making decisions that need to be thought out. No one else will live with your guilt. We are, sadly, all numbers in a giant system of papers, facts, and figures. Don't be afraid to be human and take some time to think and make good choices that won't plague your conscience or leave your loved one in a bad way. And don't be afraid to say what you think and feel to those whose job it is to plow through piles of cases—cases of people—all in a day's work to get the job done.

That is not to say these workers don't know anything. They are well trained, and you should certainly take advantage of their years of practical experience. Just keep facts and feelings separate, if at all possible, so the right steps take place and you're not faced with the two-steps-back syndrome—it'll be those steps back that wear you down and leave you gasping, grasping.

THEY SAY IT'S YOUR BIRTHDAY

It's mid-May, and the tree has budded, its leaves popping out to create shade and privacy over the Iris Street window. Laura and Anna are over for lunch, I think, and possibly one of my friends is here as well. We will be eating in the dining room, which requires only the best china serving dishes and even the silverware, if Granny has had the time to polish a gleam onto the antique spoons. The girls are busy transferring the hot food into the Royal Worchester Fine China, and I am assisting Granny in the washroom. "THEY ALWAYS REMEMBER," she sighs and smiles, "THEY ALWAYS REMEMBER ME." I nod. I know she means the girls, the little girls from across the street, all grown up now, but they are still the little girls across the street in Granny's eyes and mind. "THEY ALWAYS REMEMBER ME ON MY BIRTHDAY!"

Now, anyone who hadn't read the *Learning to Speak Alzheimer's* book would have responded, "*It's not your birthday.*" Not I. I thought, hmmm, she missed her birthday; although she was surrounded by friends and family, she was in a coma. Not wanting to burst her birthday bubble, we threw a party. We all had a blast, and Granny was thrilled beyond words. Her last words that night were to sing the praises of those girls, who would never forget her on her birthday.

Looking back, I realize that the shortcake had started the birthday train. She and Fariel had eaten fresh strawberries on sponge cake as an after-breakfast snack—Granny loves her sweets, and obviously so does Fariel. Also, adding to the charade was a birthday card from Barbara, a very fancy one I had displayed for Granny to know that Barbara was thinking of her. Barbara has faithfully written and visited for God knows how long—since she was Lenore's student—and Lenore hasn't taught in over twenty years.

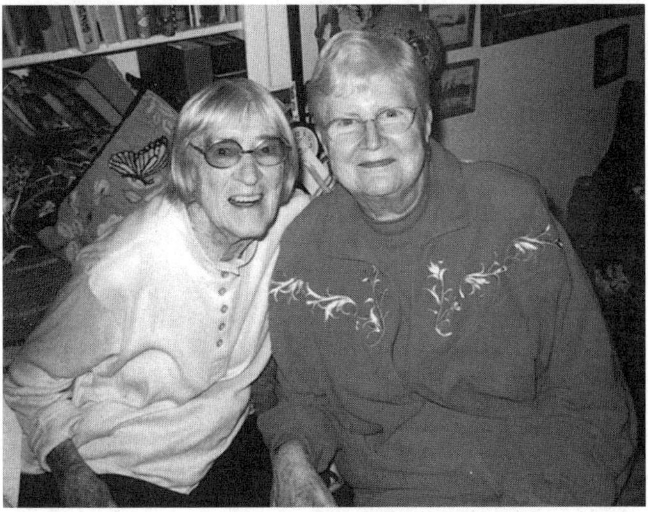

Lenore and Barbara

The next day, Granny was kind of blue. Sullen, she confides to me: "YOU'RE THE ONLY ONE WHO REMEMBERS MY BIRTHDAY."

Yikes! She's got me now! I agree to a car ride, to cheer her up. I can't bear to depress her any more by telling her that her birthday is over. This brings to light a small fact that I have yet to mention. I hate ice cream. Well, it tastes okay, but it makes me feel rather ill, so I avoid it. As you well know, Granny loves ice cream. I think she and her husband used to eat it on dates, and she and George would partake of it on their rides in the country. She loves the pleasure of eating ice cream with someone who's eating ice cream. She feels so good that she can hardly contain herself—but—she has to *pay* for the ice cream, as well as eat it with someone. She will verify the entire way home: "DID I PAY FOR THE ICE CREAM?" It's a good idea to keep the receipt for evidence, really, and it's also good to love ice cream.

So there we are, on the birthday drive, and she says, "LET'S GO FOR ICE CREAM!"

Hmmm . . . driving and writing doesn't work in city traffic—only at red lights. "IT'S MY BIRTHDAY," she reminds me before I luck out with a red light. I must be the only one on the road hoping for a red light. Oh boy, driving and avoiding ice cream can be difficult, if not impossible.

"I CAN'T BELIEVE YOU WON'T TAKE ME FOR ICE CREAM ON MY BIRTHDAY." A little guilt baffooes[1] me into Dairy Queen. She was, of course, ecstatic, and I let my aching belly be soothed by her joy.

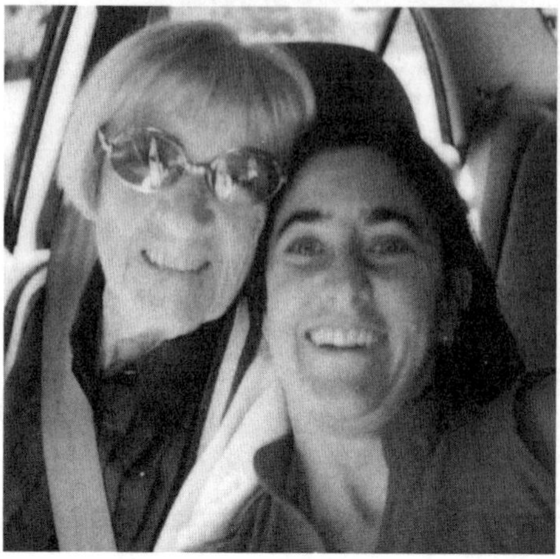

Going to meet George in Renfrew

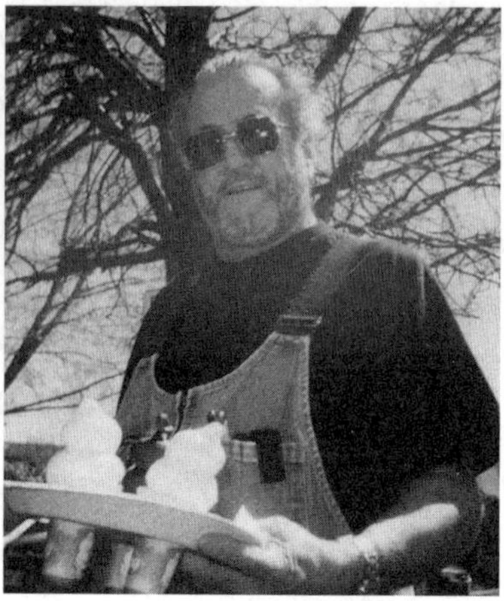

George bought us ice cream!

It literally took days and days, almost two weeks, to convince her that it wasn't her birthday. It was fun, all the celebrations, but some days she'd be terribly upset at being forgotten by the whole world on her birthday.

Ice cream is a natural remedy for Granny. Laura doesn't like ice cream either, and she taught me a trick: she smears ice cream into a glass dish and only pretends to eat it, savouring its texture as it melts in her mouth—a strange part of the job description, a white lie that creates joy. But why not?

If Granny's upset, move her from location, administer ice cream in the summer and Tetley (decaf only) in the cooler weather, and talk about the birds. As the ice cream melts, so do her worries. Both simple and effective—a drug-free prescription that can produce euphoria and calm in even the most agitated Granny.

---

[1] Baffoo: to be forced into an action to avoid shattering an altered reality.

HOLDING ON

An intimate look into the mind's eye:
I look
Eye look
I see
Eye see
The mind is a funnel or a sieve,
Or both at once,
It seems
Certain thoughts can roll
Round and round
Others, gone
Before we
Can grasp them.
Gone before our eyes
Eyes see
Eyes feel
We hold.
On we hold
Like life or death
Sometimes
If we can clasp it
Hard enough
If we clasp
When open
Our fingers
What we will see
Eye see
I see
There is nothing
My hand now
Is empty
It is all there
The emptiness
It was there
Where did it go?
What was it?
I feel it
Felt it
Miss it
Want it
I know
I knew
There was something missing
There was something
There was
Here and gone.
Not forgotten.

NO MORE HOSPITALS

Once we let go of holding on, when we realize that dying is a natural process and must be honoured as such, especially at the ripe age of ninety-three, the only conclusion to draw is that no hospital will better our last days—the food sucks and the environment is stale; not at all an appropriate place to pass on. That is our blessing: it is a commitment but a relief to know that unless Granny is to fall and break something, we will never be going back to the emergency room to waste precious hours and taxpayers' money on a diagnosis of old age.

Our palliative care practitioner makes this a possible scenario; she is available 24/7 for questions, guidance, and reassurance. Without this peace of mind, we certainly would have ended up many times at the hospital with ringing ears, seizures, minor strokes, diarrhea, and any number of other physical and mental conditions. Granny does not wish to be resuscitated—thus the DNR order—and wishes to be allowed to die in peace without electrocardiograms, wires, and hoses, where a hand to hold and pain management are the only prescriptions. I think I am strong enough for this pledge, although time will tell how I cope, when push comes to shove.

Of course, for all involved, I pray that she will depart this life quietly in her sleep, free of pain and confusion, perhaps in a dream, with the waiting arms of Evelyn and her family extended, one filled with roses and sunsets. We won't be saving Granny in any glass jars, she wishes to be scattered over the ashes of her husband, a man she loved with all her heart even through all the pain he imposed on her. I know that even after his new marriage, my grandfather, who, incidentally, committed suicide due to his manic depression—a fact that Lenore still dreads in remembering but is unable to forget—always loved Lenore. A dear friend once told me that the worst pain a human can feel is that which arises when we've wronged another human. When we see those we've wronged, we see ourselves in a mirror of shame. The strongest of personal dilemmas, shame can cause self-hate and deny us the ability to be loved, accept understanding, and trust ourselves.

In my heart, I know that Granny has forgiven Sandy for his behaviours; she understands that he struggled with mental illness, and that above it all, she will be looking for him in heaven, where he will undoubtedly be waiting to take her for a plane ride and an ice cream, beyond history, over clouds and dreams. In the heart of healing, perhaps they will return to earth to try again, together, as soulmates often do.

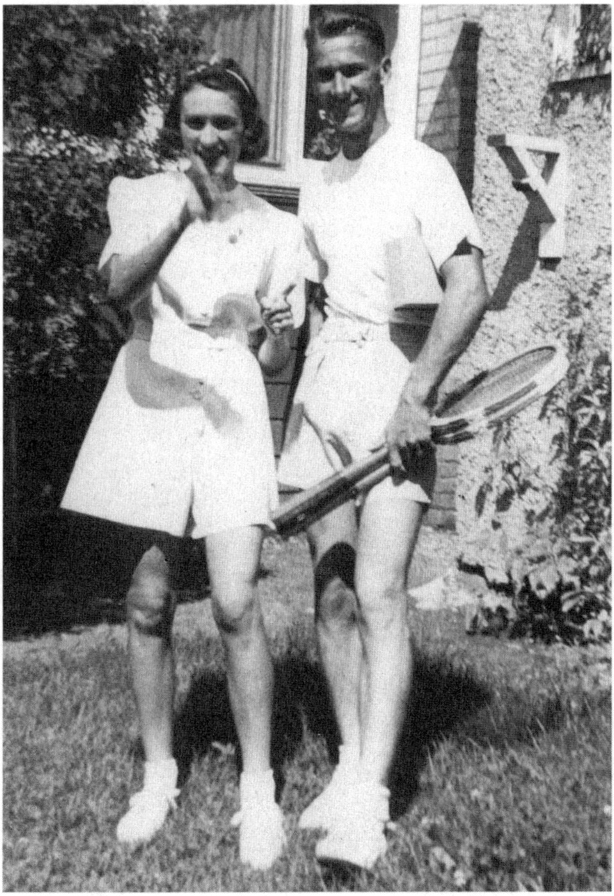

Lenore with husband, Sandy

WHERE ARE WE AT AND WHAT DO I DO

The last week has been hard on me. Perhaps it is due to my outer world infringing, these plans and commitments that keep me going, along with lack of sleep and questioning myself: "Am I doing the right things?" Of course, I'm doing my best to keep Granny comfortable and happy, an almost impossible task of late, the ringing is so intense. I can see it zap her will. Yesterday was the day she visited her brother, also the worst day of ringing I've ever seen. The pain was so great that the tears flowed freely down her face; she let me dab them dry, the effort too great for her.

Dr. Coulombe says that I'm doing a great job, which I remind myself when I have personal doubts. Should I give her the codeine? The sedative? What will help ease her tribulation without knocking her out of commission? I don't want to have to start the morphine trip again—it is so chaotic and unpredictable. Yesterday was one of those days where you look at your list of what you've given her and count the minutes until you can re-dose her with something, anything. She is uncomfortable.

"It's hell, Heather," she could barely whisper her truth. "I'm suffering," she said through tears; my tears were verging as well. I'm tired and sympathetic to the point that my head is ringing, too. Maybe I can hear her ringing, after all.

As the sedative began to work, she decided that she should lie down in her bed. Wow—this was serious. She refused lunch, too tired to eat, and fell into a deep sleep around two o'clock. Don't worry; she didn't die yesterday, although for her, it would have been a relief. I, however, thought she might; indeed, even when you're ready, the thought of death can cause a wee bit of nervous tension.

I cleaned the food cupboard and hand-oiled the hardwood floors. I am so used to saving my appetite for Granny's pleasure that I missed lunch. I didn't even notice—I will be one of those old ladies who only eat when someone's with me, to share the company more than the food. I made an apple crisp so when she awoke there would be a sweet temptation to soothe her mind and tummy, and I paced the hall, peeking in to see if she was breathing. To pass the time I played my guitar, in the hall, so I could watch from a distance, be there but give her some space of her own. I am always hovering over her—it must drive her crazy as an independent individual.

Eventually, I wake her—I don't want her to soak the bed, as she has only a day Depends™ on. She is confused about the time of day and the fact that she is wearing clothing in bed. I explain several times that she has had a nap and that it's five o'clock in the early evening. She can't grasp it. She is embarrassed that the bath lady saw her naked today. She is pretty much just upset, internally, and relatively calm on the surface. Her eyes are moving, slowing or bolting. They are still bloodshot; the pressure in her brain is pressing into her eyes. It must be torture, to say the least.

We sit together at the kitchen table with bowls of rice and chicken stir-fry.

"I DREAMT I DIED, HEATHER."

"Were you frightened?"

She nods.

"What did you see?"

"NOTHING. I WAS DEAD."

"You just knew."

"YES."

"Are you ready to go?"

"YES."

"You are a strong woman, a brave woman. I am here with you."

"ARE YOU LEAVING?"

"No, I will be here with you. Don't worry. I will always be watching over you."

"THANK YOU HEATHER. I AM AFRAID."

"Are you afraid to let go?"

"YES."

"Are you holding on for something?"

"I DON'T KNOW."

"You have done a good job with all you've done in your long life. Everything is looked after. It is okay for you to let go."

We are both a bit watery in the eyes now.

She nods again.

"I WISH I WERE DEAD."

I nod, half smiling, half teary.

"I'M AFRAID TO DIE."

She sobs, and I hold her; she is vibrating with release. I am crying, absorbing her fear and releasing mine. This isn't easy. It's beautiful but it certainly isn't easy.

"LET'S DO THE DISHES," her voice crackles, the voice of reason.

Over dessert, we continue our heartease.

"You are a wonderful woman. Thank you for everything you've done for me. You have made me, me."

"OH, HEATHER. THANK YOU. PLEASE DON'T LEAVE ME."

"I am here with you on this journey. I am blessed to be here with you. Thank you for letting me share your time."

"THANK YOU. I LOVE YOU."

"I love you. We are lucky to have each other. Thank God!"

She was awake for five hours that day, yesterday; granted, the last hours were half-awake, but filled with peace. She wanted to be with me, but was tired of holding hands. She needs the company but also the space. She likes to watch me play the guitar, so I sat and played—for her and for myself—and she drifted in and out of consciousness, with a beautiful smile on her face. She was glowing, so she was. We are growing, so we are. We are both letting go, so we must. We are experiencing a loss; we must embrace it or it will strangle us. We are gaining wisdom, a gift from beyond. Her path is getting shorter, and we must accept it. Strength and peace come from within. Love can fill our cups. Watch them as they overflow. Watch the love grow. Let love let it go. Let it go. Let's go. We're going. Going, going.

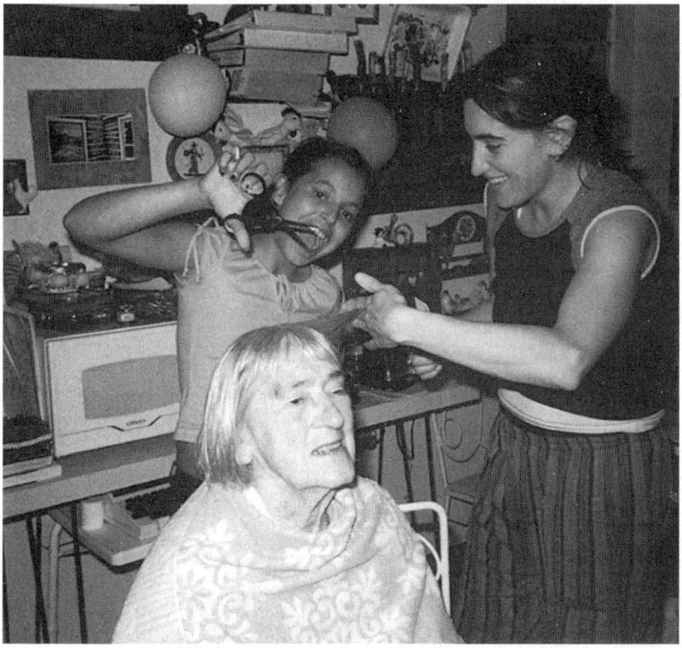

Haircut! Brittany, Heather, and Lenore

When I said that the sleepless part was the hardest part of this, I must have overlooked the emotional part, the part of you that after a night like we just had, yes, sleepless but also gut-wrenching—for lack of a better description—has left you full of thought with a clonk in your heart, a clonk like the one Hélène took home with her to Montreal. Indeed, last night and yesterday were long and unpredictable, starting with a five a.m. need to go to the bank and leading us down a hallucinogenic path, where time lines mixed together like margaritas, strong ones with more tequila than lime.

The details of these last forty-eight hours are possibly irrelevant, especially to those who do not know Lenore or the people she has talking with her in her reality. A small point of interest to you might be that Richard Nixon was here in the mid-afternoon. Until he arrived, Granny was either upset or agitated but still in reality. He woke her with his singing.

"WHO'D OF THOUGHT HE WAS SUCH A GOOD BARITONE? IT STARTED WITH A TONE, A TONE, A TONE, AND THEN THEY SANG LIKE A SONG FOR CHILDREN. IT WAS BEAUTIFUL HARMONIES. IT TOUCHED ME IN HERE," pointing to her heart. "IT ACTUALLY TOUCHED ME INSIDE! I COULD FEEL IT! DID MR. NIXON GO HOME? WITHOUT SAYING GOODBYE? I WON'T BE SEEING HIM AGAIN, I'M CERTAIN OF THAT."

We spent four hours, the kind of hours that pass without knowing, like lightning not molasses, and I learned many facts about my Granny's life that I was previously oblivious to. I found out her mother's first name, a long forgotten title—"SHE'S MOM," has been her answer for years now—and she recalled her mother's maiden name, as well. Where does this information hide? What makes it surface? As of late, Granny is no longer certain that I am her granddaughter, sometimes a cousin or a niece, sometimes "MISS" the nurse, but definitely not George's daughter. She has started to introduce us—me to my father—a highly distressing thing for him, not prepared like I am for the acceptance that she's really slipped several more rungs on the memory ladder. She accepts this new position with far greater ease than George can. I can sympathize to a point, but what can I do? I tend to laugh a lot—my prescription for release, my drug of choice.

Last night was gruelling, mostly because of the content of the night, the "what" of "who was," which has affected Granny's peace of mind. This brings me to the point of this entire chapter. You already know what Granny's behaviour is like on these dementia highs, so I needn't waste words on describing our floundering. I had quite a bit of time to let thoughts run through my head between getting up and down all night. One thought was of a note I had left for Laura, Betty, and Hélène when I was away in August: "**DON'T GO THROUGH A CRISIS ALONE.**" I'd even written it bold and large. I can't possibly expect anyone to go through this alone, but then you find yourself wondering in the middle of the night whom to call.

Whom do you call?

I also wondered to myself, where can I go to get some sleep, tomorrow?

I'm taking my time getting to this point; it is evasive and a bit blurry yet. So, last night was a personal experience for me. I understood what Granny was going through and listened from the rock I stand on—the stone I try to sleep on—but I just can't seem to get comfortable. It is bedrock, it goes way down deep, and I think it runs parallel with the earth, curving and undulating just below the surface, folding over like caramel.

It is important to remember that rock was once a flowing liquid, before it moulded itself over and around the earth's core. It is the ground we stand on that is passed on through generations; they call it cultural diffusion—that is, non-physical inherent traits, attitudes, emotions, fears, and thought patterns. These are qualities that as individuals we might want to enhance (the positive ones), and others we shall wish to overcome, once we realize their presence in our lives, which is more often than not the challenge: REALIZING. We are conceivably oblivious to that which is normal to us. That is what "coming of age" entails, a forgotten destiny for our culture. We become adults, and are expected to become independent—financially and physically—and no expectations are placed on evolving into higher beings. The word "enlightenment" is hardly ever spoken in regard to the responsibility of human advancement. As the fly on the wall these past hours, I've acquired new insights, experienced yet another aspect of Granny's life and personality, shedding light onto my world, a world that has developed at times from outside influences, beyond my control. It hit close to home and has left me with ponderous enlightenments, in respect to my own cultural diffusion.

This whole rock analogy brings to mind an expression I once read, "May all your obstacles in life be stepping stones, rather than stumbling blocks." Adversity is a gift to overcome. It is stepping stones if you wish or toe-catchers if you stumble. We can't conquer rocks and probably shouldn't waste time trying to—you can step on them, over them, or skirt your way around them. You can also chisel them into smaller rocks, pocket-sized if you feel the need to carry them around with you. You can, by all means, put your back into it and heave, HO! that boulder, down big hills, over cliffs and into deep bodies of water—out of sight but never out of mind.

What I am getting to, this elusive point that has been tickling at me until I've had these moments to write—I'm letting it jell into form while Fariel sits with Granny—two days after the hallucinations started, one day after we started to tranquilize her, seven hours after she has fallen into an unwakable slumber of huffing breaths that stop—and there is nothing—for sometimes half a minute before recommencing.

Coincidentally, I am reading a narrative story about a young girl who is finding herself, her roots. She is coming of age, and is forced to *unlearn*—the most important aspect, I think, of becoming human and conscious. The book has come to me at a good time, offering a sense of higher knowing just when I need reassurance.

Granny has managed to unlearn by example and personal realization much of what she was taught—by example, I presume. The parts that are haunting her are the parts she's held onto, these rocks and pebbles in her pockets and shoes, these boulders submersed under dark waters. Finding them now is half the trouble—throwing even the littlest stones takes a lot of mental effort when you're at death's door. The Buddhists believe that when you die, your soul goes to a place of limbo where your essence awaits rebirth. It is a time of quiet contemplation for those who are clean from the burdens of living, a floating, peaceful reality; unless of course you are full of fears and unresolved anxieties. The more a spirit has released its fears, the less power these demons have to force the soul to return to earth in haste, perhaps making an inappropriate choice for the next life.

It doesn't matter if you believe in reincarnation, or if I do, for that matter. Almost all cultures have their own beliefs, but a common thread runs through human spirituality: as death draws near, we want to release ourselves from the burdens of baggage, the wrongs done—we seek forgiveness and offer it. We seek a clean slate, an empty palette. Rather than wait until the bitter end, I can see that it is best to let go, as we go, to forgive on the path as we walk it, instead of struggling to get back to the crossroads passed, in order to liberate our minds, hearts, and souls.

Let this be an invitation for you to set free that which burdens you, accepting that everything in life happens for the higher good, offering gifts and lessons if we are wise enough to see and arise to the challenge of understanding. So, at this time, I have learned a lot about where I came from, what strings pulled the puppets of my ancestors and the underlying attitudes that prevailed. Hooks embedded are difficult to remove, and unfortunately for my granny, these barbs are holding on tight. She is fighting to let them go, one by one, because they are keeping her trapped in this realm, suffering. I'm certain that she knows she must be free before she passes, and will continue this soul work until the job is done. I am blessed to be a part—well, not an active part but a silent witness to her healing.

That is the bottom line to this whole rattling dissertation—our society generally allows strangers to witness and aid loved ones through this path of passage, either in hospitals or nursing homes. I understand the pain of seeing these tribulations; first-hand insight has been granted to me as a gift, one that many will avoid due to fear and miss the keys they hold, the keys of release. It is this trepidation that keeps society on the physical plane rather than a spiritual one, hence halting the evolution process, keeping individuals from realizing and releasing old rocks, or climbing up onto them—and the view is always a lot better from the top. Perspective can lend beauty and wisdom to adversity. Resolution creates resiliency, thus we can carry with us our strengths—a far easier chore than carting around rocks; yes, indeed, it is a far easier fate.

LET'S LET GO

All I can say is that Granny is a beautiful woman. She has graced everyone she meets, sharing herself and her light of being. I'm sure she has carried her weight on her shoulders, but she also must have let go of a great many things, certainly giving openly and spreading joy.

We were speaking about heaven and hell. It's no wonder that she is afraid to die—she thinks she is going to hell because she's had such a hard life. My heart goes to her. My heart *is* her, at times.

It's difficult to pray for someone you love so dearly, to let go. It is only humane—that's human—psyche, emotional body, etheric field, the rope that ties us from the deepest roots of the earth into the heavens—but it is still terribly hard. Grieving is a natural process. I am experiencing a long, drawn-out grief for the loss of Granny. I love all of who she is, and that includes who she was and who she grew to be. I think that the more we let go of in this lifetime, the lighter we will go. Let's let go. The more let go, the more room to grow, to glow, let's. We glow from the inside out, let us glow. We can sense it, even see it. We shine, let's go, let's glow. If we hold nothing we have nothing to lose, let's let go. Hold my hand, and I will be holding, too, let's go. In my heart forever, let's go. We two shall wander; yes, let's let go.

DOING IT AS BEST I CAN

You know that being with Granny is a beautiful thing. Granted, it is a full-on job in many ways—I always have an ear open—but the main objective is to keep her safe and as happy as possible, even with ringing ears and aching bones.

For me, it is a fine line, this balance between being and doing: being for me, being for her, doing for me and, naturally, doing for her. And what's more, letting her do for herself, allowing for independence; even if it takes five times as long to complete a chore, so be it. We are certainly not in any races here, and not about to start any, either. It is how it is, and is much easier if I don't expect to get much of anything done for myself. Personal time has become a luxury and a bonus, a sacred place that I cherish when it arises. That is the entire catch: it's probably worse to know the catch than to ignore it, because the further I get from my self and my wants, the less energy I have for her.

That is why respite is all too important—beyond importance; it is a necessity. Once a caregiver can find the help she or he needs to have the space—and by space I mean peace of mind and allowance for his or her own life—the space fills itself. It is a giant circle, a cycle of existence that gets easier and easier once we actually isolate our own needs. I'm speculating a bit here, drawing from my own struggles and awareness, in my determination of the importance of keeping myself centred, inspired, and socially active.

When I am happy, it is easy, easy like a breeze, to keep Granny happy. To balance the scale, her happiness makes me happy, too. It is a two-way street, this care partnership. Although helping and sharing brings me joy, it doesn't fill my needs and sometimes even empties them to the point of hollow. You could probably hear the echo some days, the reverberation of ideas in my mind, rattling about without the spark to initiate, let alone complete, them. I have to remind myself that I am doing something: a simple something that is a major something, a something that is far more important than anything I could ever hold in my hands, something that I will hold forever in my heart of hearts.

I now know to reach for help when I am exhausted. I no longer wait until I'm too tired to even reach, and that took a while to learn. I like to think of myself as a rock, sturdy and proud—not stubborn and heavy—but all good things have their flip side and I'm the first to admit that fact. I will also admit that the rock I am can get stuck, hung up in the tundra of adversity. Perhaps I am as stubborn as Granny, an inherent trait of inescapable determination to stand strong, long—even alone, if need be.

Hopefully I have graduated from this blind resolve, and will in the future see the boundaries that keep us in the realm of coping instead of drowning in circumstance. Like I've said before, getting help is the only way to go. No one can be everything to anyone, not even for ourselves, even if we're used to standing alone in high winds, with hail, on a fine line. If the margin is narrow, we are all sure to fall, sooner than later.

All the support we have received and accepted has widened my margin and strengthened my fences. I can now see farther, clearer, and with less effort. My pride is never sacrificed in accepting or asking for their help; it is foolish to think it would be, but we all think foolishly sometimes. And what's more, Granny's time here is a gift, and not a gift solely for me, either. I can see the joy she shares—it cultivates itself and miraculously grows within those who give themselves to give.

It is easy, when you're in this position I am in, to lose track of yourself. It's not something that you can follow, like a rabbit in the forest, because it is little things that disappear with no trace. You can't fight it, either, because that would require effort that you might not have the energy for. Perspective is everything. Even a little time away can renew my energy and I can get back on the path to and of myself, without seeking old tracks to know the way.

The craziest thing is that for an unseasoned caregiver, when they do get away, it feels like they are *running away*. They probably are, too, especially if someone has tried to hit you on your way out to go dancing because you "certainly don't love me if you're going out without me!"

Catch 22, on the scene! You feel like you're abandoning your partner; however, you've been abandoning yourself. Guilt . . . guilty of guilt, we caregivers must let it all go and lie down in the battlefield and admit that we aren't capable of abandoning ourselves to be there for someone else. We have to wander without worry. It took me months to finally leave without worry in my heart and mind.

Let me be perfectly blunt: if she dies . . . she dies. Whether or not I am there, nothing will bring her back; the other side of the coin being that if she doesn't die, will I get those moments back? Let's face it, there have been so many instances of *this could be it, Heather* that after awhile you're ready for it.

You know what it is—we all have different beliefs, but we all know it is called death. People die. Trees die. Seasons change. It's inevitable. Something profound happens and it's a beautiful thing, a rite of passage, especially for those who die of old age. Quite honestly, Granny has had lots of time to prepare for this journey. She's ready . . . set, go! She says almost every night, "I HOPE I DON'T WAKE UP!" or "WOULD YOU JUST KILL ME?" like a bedtime prayer. I wish for her the peace she needs to move on.

So, caregivers everywhere, ask yourself:

Who is to blame if I give up a dream for this cause? Would my partner wish me this sacrifice of myself? How do we give *of* ourselves and *to* ourselves all in the same breath? How do we step away and give only to ourselves?

Now admit to yourself:

I am, of course, the only one controlling me and I will soar (and at times flounder) happily and consciously, creating this delicate meshing between being a caregiver and an individual. Three cheers for intention! Four cheers for achieving! Five for enduring! Six for resilience and one for the hell of it! Sound your wild YAWP! even if and especially only for yourself to hear.

I hate to brag, but I think I have finally got it figured out, to a point. I have taken all these lessons, yes, those quiet lingering ones, and made a foundation to create and rejoice from. I can say that my ship has become evenly keeled, with an inner balance of practised calm and patience.

I remind myself that it is okay to grieve. Tears are clean and they can wash away a lot of what holds us down, even that which we cannot see. Our boundaries can be flexible, as I am learning, in many and all areas of our lives. I find myself sometimes withdrawing from certain aspects of life, mostly because I'm afraid of any major waves or storm fronts hitting, crashing over my bow. That is what I have to learn next, I guess: that sometimes these waves can benefit the hull, washing it down. All in good time, all in good time.

I am supposed to think about the future. My friends keep saying things like, "Guess you're in it for the long haul."

I guess so, too. Yes, indeed, it's probably true. I hope to be by her side when she passes, although I think I may keep her holding on. Cliché.

So, I remind myself every day, that everything will happen as it should; that things materialize as we need them. I think I'm still pretty much as sane as I've always been, maybe even more so—certainly more grounded in a far-out way. I try and see the things I've learned, remember them, and live them. I am fortunate enough to be able to bend in these wild winds that drive the sails of our boat. I am even able to control these gusts and direct them so they work with us instead of fighting, tacking back and forth to go nowhere.

I can keep an old lady happy, in her home, where she wants to be.

I can make myself happy, too, in an old lady's home, where I want to be.

If heaven can wait, then I guess it can wait a little bit longer.

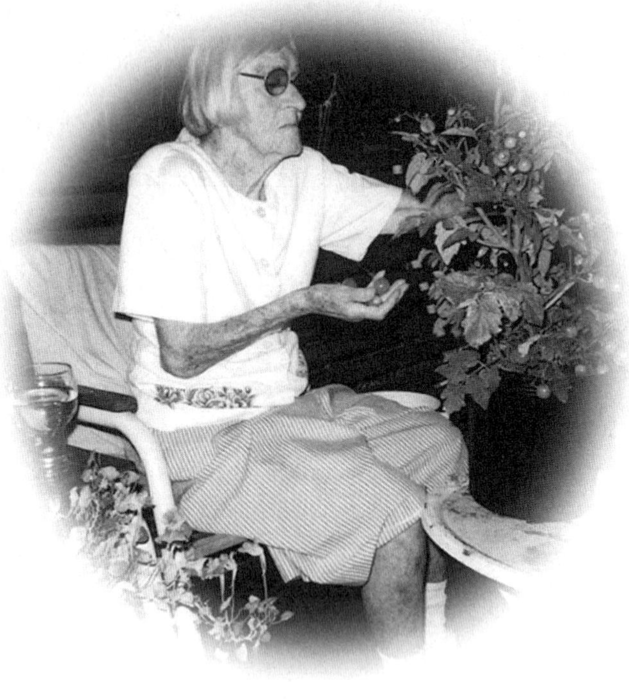

Harvesting tomatoes

ABOUT THE AUTHOR

Deedee was raised on an Ottawa Valley farm at the end of a long dirt road, where she learned to entertain herself with nature, art, and music. She makes her path through the sanctity of the northern forest, drawing inspiration both from within and from the beauty that surrounds her to create vivid and vibrant paintings.

Deedee lives off the grid in a quaint home near Wilno, Ontario, where she is working on her second book.

To order more copies of

If Heaven Can Wait...

Finding Grace through Alzheimer's

Deedee Sanderson

Contact:

GENERAL STORE PUBLISHING HOUSE

499 O'Brien Road, Box 415
Renfrew, Ontario Canada K7V 4A6
Telephone: 1-800-465-6072
Fax: (613) 432-7184
www.gsph.com

VISA and MASTERCARD accepted.